HOW TO DRAG A BODY *and* OTHER SAFETY TIPS YOU HOPE TO NEVER NEED

Also by Judith Matloff

Home Girl

No Friends but the Mountains

Fragments of a Forgotten War

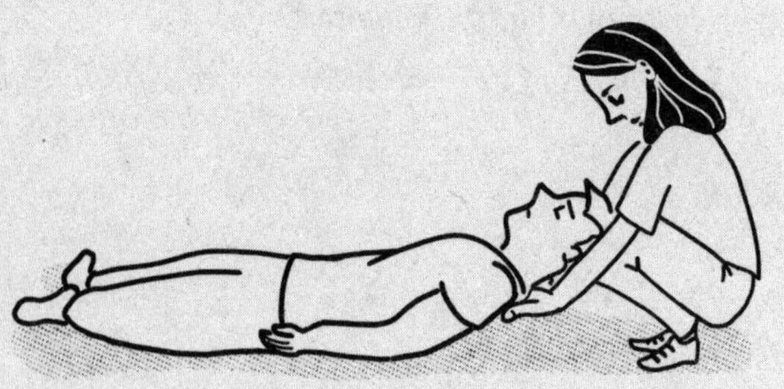

HOW TO DRAG A BODY *and* OTHER SAFETY TIPS YOU HOPE TO NEVER NEED

SURVIVAL TRICKS FOR HACKING, HURRICANES, AND HAZARDS LIFE MIGHT THROW AT YOU

JUDITH MATLOFF

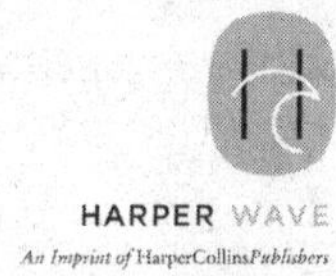

HARPER WAVE
An Imprint of HarperCollins*Publishers*

This book contains advice and information relating to health care. It should be used to supplement rather than replace the advice of your doctor or another trained health professional. If you know or suspect that you have a health problem, it is recommended that you seek your physician's advice before embarking on any medical program or treatment. All efforts have been made to assure the accuracy of the information contained in this book as of the date of publication. The publisher and the author disclaim liability for any medical outcomes that may occur as a result of applying the methods suggested in this book.

HarperCollins books may be purchased for educational, business, or sales promotional use. For information, please email the Special Markets Department at SPsales@harpercollins.com.

FIRST EDITION

Designed by Bonni Leon-Berman
Illustrations by Sharon Levy

Library of Congress Cataloging-in-Publication Data has been applied for.
ISBN 978-0-06-297093-0

20 21 22 23 24 LSC 10 9 8 7 6 5 4 3 2 1

In memory of my mother

CONTENTS

HOW TO DRAG A BODY *and* OTHER SAFETY TIPS YOU HOPE TO NEVER NEED

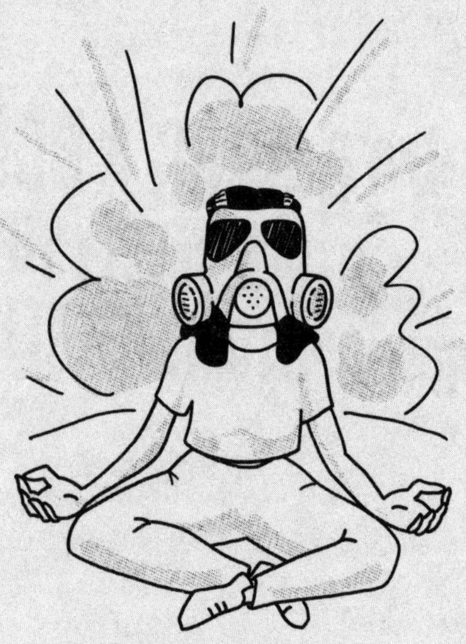

EVERYTHING'S FINE

Chapter 1

THE POWER OF PLANNING

The seeds of this book sprouted in 1992, when I made some really stupid mistakes.

I was working as a correspondent for the Reuters news agency when my boss sent me to Angola, a notoriously tumultuous African country. I was supposed to report on its first democratic elections. Until then, I had covered the odd riot, but I generally did business reporting or press conferences, where the biggest danger was being pushed out of the way by an aggressive cameraman trying to get a better shot.

Now I was in Angola. For thirty-five years a relentless civil war there had killed millions of people and left land mines strewn all over the country. Peace had been hastily negotiated just months before my arrival, but no one was sure it would last. Armed guerrillas were roaming around the country under the leadership of Jonas Savimbi, a venal sociopath known to burn people alive. He was the sort of guy who raped underlings' wives and starved entire towns because he didn't like their party politics. Savimbi had already made clear that he *had* to become president. For some reason my bosses and I hadn't considered what might happen if he didn't. After all, he was an egomaniac. Well, Savimbi lost the elections. In response, he ordered his men to pick up their rocket-propelled grenade launchers and go door-to-door to round up critics. Suddenly, roadblocks popped up on my way to interviews, and a car bomb exploded and shooting erupted near my hotel. I was clueless about these new working conditions and actually thought one should run *toward* heavy-caliber machine-gun exchanges to see what was going on rather than cower at a safe distance. My only previous experience with battle was watching World War II movies with my father, who once showed me the Mauser rifle he had lifted from a dead soldier. I had no idea how it worked. That was the extent of it.

It's amazing that I got out of Angola in one piece. I did dumb things, like naïvely stroll through a mine dump filled with smoking shells. It didn't occur to me that my leg could be blown off if I stepped on the wrong spot. I had also packed the wrong malaria medication and got a 102-degree fever that lasted for days. When I recovered, Savimbi's number two came to my hotel lobby to tell me that he didn't appreciate my reporting. "You're not writing positive things about us," he said. Gripping my wrist in his fish-cold hand, he warned me to leave town "or else." I wasted valuable days deliberating how to respond to this death threat, and by the time I finally decided to make a dash for the airport, the fighting had spread to the tarmac and all flights out were canceled. Rebels, meanwhile, had thoughtfully mined roads and blown up bridges, so driving across the nearest border wasn't an option, either. Stuck in the capital, Luanda, I strayed into a courtyard of snipers and nearly got shot in the forehead. I also wasn't dressed for success—success being survival—and scurried about in flimsy Keds. Flak jackets? Never heard of 'em. Finally, I sabotaged my only communication with the outside world, the ten-thousand-dollar satellite phone my editor had given me, one of a mere handful in town, when I failed to plug in a surge protector during one of the constant blackouts. The phone had to go to a repair shop, and there wasn't one in all of Angola. Lest you think I was a complete fool, let me say that such ignorance was common in those days. At that time, the news business didn't have safety protocols. We simply headed to a sketchy area with a bottle of Bell's whisky and cries of "Good luck!" The office would rejoice if you came back intact. If you didn't, the boss would hold a memorial and send flowers to your family. If you were really popular, someone would open a single malt and pass it around the newsroom.

Eventually, the man who wanted to execute me was shot in the legs (not by me), so I didn't have to worry about him anymore, and battles at the airport stopped long enough for commercial flights to resume. On the plane back to Johannesburg, where I'd been living for the past year, I ordered a sparkling brut to celebrate the safe exit. But I had a nagging suspicion that with some simple homework and forethought, I could have operated in a more prudent manner.

That conviction grew deeper as my career unfolded over the next few decades, on five continents. I've since reported on seven civil wars, one genocide, several separatist rebellions, and forty-eight assorted rogue militias, gangs, vigilantes, and drug cartels. The civil unrest and mob situations

I covered probably number in the hundreds. As time went on, equipping myself with contingency plans and risk analyses, I felt more confident going into other problematic situations, like landslides and gloomy American neighborhoods and middle school soccer games. I learned how to negotiate with armed drunk teenagers at foreign checkpoints and to search under my Citi Golf for explosives. I discovered how to stay reasonably clean in a shelter and how to apply pressure to a spurting artery. I gleaned how to protect my phone conversations from Vladimir Putin's intelligence agents and outwit policemen bent on rape.

As Confucius once said, "He who fails to prepare, prepares to fail." Or as I like to say, "Without proper planning, you're screwed."

I got into media safety training in 2005, after too many colleagues were maimed, raped, killed, or kidnapped. I had faced too many close calls myself, and it occurred to me, and others in the industry, that popping cheap airplane champagne after surviving wasn't an effective tactic. We needed to lessen the odds of fatality by guarding against the perils. To that end, I incorporated new safety protocols into my classes at Columbia University's Graduate School of Journalism, where I've been teaching for nearly two decades. Workshops that I ran outside the university blossomed into a consulting business for organizations around the world. And as one of the few women who did safety training, I honed primers that addressed the special needs of females.

As my clientele grew, people began to approach me outside the small journalist community. Most of them were women, who felt particularly exposed to danger and unsure how to react. There was a college junior who was spending a gap year in Jordan and wanted to know what precautions she should take. Someone who was vacationing in Puerto Rico during hurricane season asked about generators and contracting Zika while pregnant. Everyone wanted to know about preparing for the surge of natural disasters that have been hitting lately. In 2017, after a gunman massacred fifty-eight people at a music festival in Las Vegas, I received a torrent of emails from acquaintances, some of whom I barely knew. They wanted ballistic advice in case they faced similar situations. Should they run bent over in a zigzag pattern, like in the movies? (Answer: That depends.) Should they fashion tourniquets from belts? (Negative.) Where was the safest place to sit at stadiums? (Near an exit.) Should they no longer take kids to concerts?

Their questions are reasonable, considering that more than four hundred Americans perished from mass shootings in 2019 alone. Random citizens have been slaughtered in schools, nightclubs, churches, and streets. Demonstrations are increasingly turning violent, even fatal. Recent events have taught us that everyone, from neighbors to postal workers, should know how to identify a pipe bomb. Experience with violence is no longer limited to the few of us who report on exotic wars and crises overseas.

How to deal with active shooters and homemade explosives and being teargassed at a protest are just a fraction of the questions I receive on a regular basis. One man asked if his eleven-year-old niece should carry a knife on the subway. (No!) Women inquire about how to prevent sexual coercion in the age of #MeToo. In light of the Equifax hack, credit card holders beg for digital tips to secure financial transactions. And everyone wants to know how to handle a stampede at Walmart on Black Friday.

This book arose from those conversations.

Many professions routinely prepare for emergencies and accidents—the military, first responders, and fund managers, to name a few. Law professors teach the worst-case method in classes. Doctors get ready for the "just-in-case scenario" when they order a battery of tests. Regular folks do the same on a daily basis, like when we buy life insurance or sign a prenuptial agreement. "Be Prepared" is the motto of many professional organizations, and even of the Girl Scouts. It should be every citizen's, too. That slogan means we should think about and also rehearse how to act during a crisis. Preparedness helps you manage the risks and make calmer decisions because you've already thought them through. It's critical to your processing information—information that is constantly changing—in that instant of panic. You don't have time to reflect during a tornado; you need to act quickly and with certainty. With that self-assurance comes agency.

Contrary to popular assumptions, imagining the dire consequences of a given crisis and then strategizing to mitigate them actually creates a greater sense of confidence. And research shows that specific training for particular events enhances a feeling of mastery in other situations.

Being skilled and forward-thinking is potentially lifesaving. Flight attendants on airplanes gesticulate toward the oxygen mask, but how many of us pay attention? If you're in a plane crash and have scoped the exits and paid attention, you have a 50 percent greater chance of survival. If debris from a blown engine smashes a window and causes a drop in cabin pressure, you'll regret that you didn't watch. That happened during a Southwest flight, and a passenger died. It could have been any of us.

You can't control terrifying events, but you can be ready for them.

This book will cover pretty much any eventuality you might face, be it a violent protest, a live shooter, emergency first aid, a terrorist attack, a natural disaster, social media harassment, or emotional fallout from an upsetting event. Some of the situations I describe might seem extreme, but others are surprisingly commonplace—a safe haven during a severe storm, protective garb for protests, and how to talk to kids about scary events, to name a few.

No matter what you're up against, the guiding principles are the same, as is the goal: to build self-assurance so that you're not at the mercy of in-the-moment reactions and fear. Preparedness is about preserving agency via exit routes, mental or physical. It's about mastering situational awareness in a nonparanoid and healthy way and gearing up psychologically and literally by having the right tools at the ready.

My aim is that you'll be prepared for the rare event, not that you'll need to apply the wisdom contained in every chapter. It'd be unfortunate to have a brush with, for example, identity theft, radiation, mudslides, active shooters, riots, and a harassing boss, one after another. But you'll likely stumble into at least a few of the scenarios in this book, or worry about their occurring. At the least, you should know what to do just in case. For good measure, I've added more quotidian tips, including first aid and how to pack and dress for maximum safety, which we war reporters know how to do with our eyes closed.

This guide is geared toward both men and women, but with an emphasis on the latter. Women are more likely to be groped, raped, stalked, harassed online, and to die in a hurricane. But that doesn't mean men don't need to prepare for natural disasters or violence as much as their higher-risk peers. Men should consult the manual, too. The tips are meant to calibrate anyone's thinking to best deal with stressful situations.

Maybe you attend protests where brawls could break out.

Perhaps you live in an earthquake zone and need to assemble an emergency kit.

Maybe you want to build emotional resilience before, during, and after a serious car accident.

Perhaps you're a college student worried about date rape at fraternity parties.

Possibly you're in a profession that sends you to crisis zones.

I hope you will find this book inviting, demystifying, and also comforting and helpful. The Resources section at the back offers leads on more information and training. Being skilled and forward-thinking is reassuring as well as potentially lifesaving.

One last thing. Don't let statistics about female vulnerability alarm you. As a five-foot-three-and-a-quarter-inch woman who weighs less than a bag of cement, I've learned a few things. Namely, that attitude and mind-set are priceless for overcoming adversity. What Alexander Graham Bell once said applies to everyone, from war correspondents to high school sophomores: “Before anything else, preparation is the key to success.”

SOME BASICS

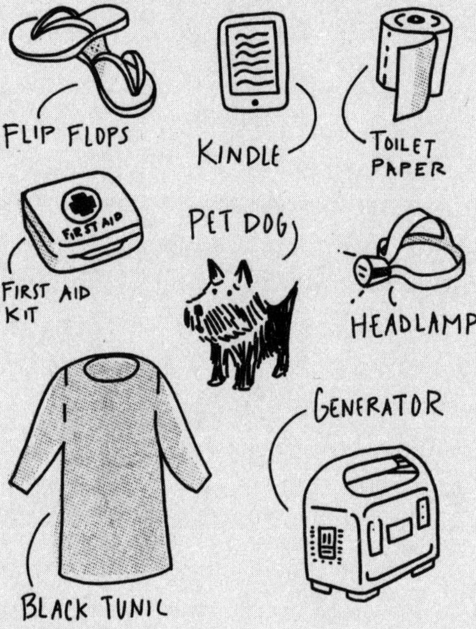

FLIP FLOPS
KINDLE
TOILET PAPER
FIRST AID
FIRST AID KIT
PET DOG
HEADLAMP
GENERATOR
BLACK TUNIC

Chapter 2

THE BASICS

Think of this book as an operating manual for whatever hazards life throws at you. It's a *What to Expect When You're Expecting*, except instead of awaiting a six-pound bundle of joy, you're preparing for some kind of man-made or natural disaster. You can flip to the section that applies to your particular concern (say, a tsunami or travel), or you can go step by step, calamity by calamity. All the knowledge is lifesaving and applicable no matter where you live in the world. The idea is to help you feel in control, rather than freaked out. And it's easy to feel freaked out; the world is anxiety-producing. So, it's best to prepare yourself as much as possible.

Still, no matter how well prepared you think you are, the reality is that you might end up in situations where you have to eke it out by the skin of your teeth or with the help of your guardian angel. I'm here to guide you to the happy medium, which is learning how to reasonably predict outcomes and get ready for them. Psychologists have a term for this: *planful problem solving*. Every woman who has ever carried a tote bag filled with diapers, Cheerios, stickers, and stuffed animals is familiar with the concept. You know what you (and others) are likely to run into, and you try to account for those eventualities.

Yet, you can't be a walking ball of anxiety all the time. So, in order to achieve the maximum Zen attitude in the face of adversity, I'm suggesting you strategize like a war correspondent. Half of effective war correspondence involves logistics—planning where to go, when to go, how to go; knowing how to thrive once you're there; and then getting home still breathing and with all your fingers and feet and organs still attached. To maximize a successful outcome, you need to make thought-out choices and mentally accept what an emergency might look like if life goes sideways.

To begin, look at the big picture of a given situation and ask yourself, What's my game plan? The answer depends on how you respond to four questions: (1) What's my exit strategy? (2) Whom do I reach in case of emergency? (3) What's the realistic worst-case scenario, and how can I mitigate that outcome? And finally, (4) What do I do if none of this works?

The next layer of questions looks like this:

- Whom do I tell when I'm traveling, at a riot, or hunkering down in a storm? (Family, lawyer, coworkers?)
- What personal affairs do I put in order before an event? (Do I make a list of contact numbers, buy protective software, create a will?)
- What should I know before going to another country or attending a protest? (A lot.)
- What equipment do I need? (Do I have shelter, food, water, medical supplies, the right clothing, and relevant documents?)

Before traveling to a conflict zone, reporters are advised to create a guide for themselves and an appointed proxy to follow to ensure their safe return. We fill out two forms, one for crisis communications and the other for risk assessment. The key to completing them is not necessarily knowing all the answers, but knowing *where* to find them and who has authority regarding a given topic. To use a real-world, non-crisis example, say I'm having an issue with my iPhone signal. Who's in charge? Who's the keeper of this knowledge? Is it Apple, or the building I'm in? If the latter, is there too much concrete in the wall? If so, whom do I contact to fix it? T-Mobile? Can I troubleshoot by searching online? Google is my go-to when the answer's not obvious, and from there I figure out who would best serve me. The same line of questioning applies to a crisis. News reports predict a hard rain's gonna fall. Who can advise me on evacuating? Would it be the local authorities or the National Weather Service? (Answer: Both.) How do I board up windows? (Consult a DIY site.)

I'll give guidance with specificity in each chapter. Rest assured that figuring this out will become second nature over time. Like any skill set, it just takes practice.

RISK ANALYSIS FORM

The essential document you should keep on hand is a risk analysis form. This outlines the perils you might face and suggests ways to mitigate or prevent them. A sample risk analysis form used widely among journalists looks like this:

Circle any of the following risks you may face:

Abduction/kidnapping

Abusive authorities

Armed conflict

Carjacking

Electronic harassment

Environmental contamination

Gangs

Home/office invasion

Identity theft

Infectious diseases

Land mines

Mass shooting/cross fire

Natural disasters and extreme weather

Nuclear strike

Petty crime/theft

Physical and/or electronic surveillance

Political instability

PTSD

Radiation/contamination

Riots/demonstrations

Road/air/boat accidents

Sexual assault

Sexual harassment

Stalking, hacking

Terrorist attack

Violent and organized crime

War

To get you started, these three examples range in gravity from "meh" to serious. Each one comes with a clear set of actions that can be taken.

1. Misadventure when walking the dog
How serious: Not very

How likely: Very

Risks: Step in poop, forget plastic bag, get hit by an electric bicycle, provoke Rottweiler twice your dog's size

Measures: Pack wet wipes to clean shoe. Keep plastic bags with leash. Don't walk with your nose in cell phone. Stride with confidence when walking by Rottweiler. Do not show fear.

2. Attack during a concert

How serious: Very

How likely: Random

Risks: Death, mutilation, losing a limb, suffocation in a stampede, not getting a refund for a ticket, psychological trauma

Measures: Sit by an exit. Wear easy-to-run-in laced boots. Avoid concerts entirely. Learn to stanch bleeding with Stop the Bleed (see Resources). Check fine print for refunds. Stand sideways in stampede.

3. Broken leg while hiking during flash flood

How serious: Depends on remoteness

How likely: Depends on location

Risks: Stranded for days, long-term health complications, death by exposure

Measures: Don't hike alone. Carry beacons. Turn on GPS. Let others know your route. Check weather advisories beforehand. Know how to set fractures. Identify nearest hospital. Carry health insurance card and ID. Pack extra water/food, painkillers, a flashlight, and a jacket. Don't stray off path. Take a survival course.

This is how I went about doing a risk analysis for a recent trip to Zion National Park in Utah. First, I called my friend Abby, who has trekked there many a time. She thought my husband and I were nuts to go during a 108-degree heat wave, but we'd booked the vacation well in advance, and no one had anticipated such a high temperature. She suggested we escape the worst of the heat with early-morning and late-afternoon walks. She also warned us about a trail known as the Narrows, a flash flood mecca from which there's no escape route. This was prime flash flood season. Sufficiently alarmed about exposure, I went to an accredited medical website to look for protection. Easy peasy: loose clothes, hydration, wide-brimmed hat, seek shade. Then I went to the park's website to learn about other local dangers besides scorching sun and flash floods. The site revealed plenty of other things to worry about: rock falls, rattlesnakes, and one particularly treacherous trail called Angels Landing, where ten hikers had plunged to their deaths in recent years. Note to self: Being a clumsy person with severe vertigo, skip the treacherous trail and opt for easier ones where no one has died, at least not yet. Even on the gentler paths, we'd need an escape route in case one of us twisted an ankle or collapsed from the heat. I also knew that cell reception would be spotty on the trails, but I figured that one of the millions of other hikers could make it down to the visitor center to call for help. Or my strong husband could lug me in his arms. On the recommendation of the experienced Abby, I also slathered on sunscreen, arranged the aforementioned heat protection, and brought along sturdy footwear, dried peaches, and maps.

One should always update the plan, of course. A quick

check-in with rangers when we arrived revealed that no rain was expected for days, so we didn't worry about flash floods or ponchos. But they cautioned against venomous rattlesnakes, which were crawling out from under rocks to search for ever-scarcer rodents. The deadly serpents have a strike distance of a few feet, the rangers warned, so we should give them a wide berth in case of an encounter.

Sure enough, a fat rattler about three feet long blocked my descent one day. The reptile was napping in the sun and wouldn't give way to tourists stomping about. He just stayed put. Along came three excited Frenchwomen who apparently hadn't gotten the rattlesnake memo and leaned in close to take selfies. The creature flicked its tail ominously. Then an elderly man approached and thumped his walking stick on the ground to get the snake to move—again, not a wise approach, as I had learned during my research about serpents, because vibrations provoke rattlers to attack. Mitigation time! I edged backward, about six feet away from it, until the viper eventually slithered off. And I henceforth steered clear of excited Frenchwomen and elderly men bearing walking sticks on the path.

In case you hunger for more examples, here's a disaster-related one using the same principles.

At the turn of the last century, the internet was abuzz with fears of a software glitch dubbed Y2K that risked stopping computer systems from rolling from 1999 to 2000. Such a programming failure could affect power grids and even nuclear reactors, so the worst-case scenario went. My husband and I were living in Moscow at the time, where the Chernobyl meltdown was fresh in everyone's mind. We didn't trust the Russian government to update its creaky computers or give the public a straight answer. Western diplomats couldn't advise us as to what to expect from the unreliable Ruskies and recommended we celebrate New Year's Eve far, far away. However, as bureau chief, I felt duty-bound to remain in town to take care of the staff during a potential catastrophe.

My husband and I moved into mitigation. We stockpiled enough food and water for two weeks, dry and canned stuff that could be eaten raw in case the gas stove and fridge failed. The pantry heaved with supplies, including extra toilet paper, lighters, candles, and batteries for flashlights and radios. We filled up the tub in case the water system broke down. A generous friend accumulated iodine pills for a big group in case of radiation poisoning. Family and employers back in the States were alerted to reach one another if news emerged of a meltdown. We powered up the satellite phone, which would operate if the cell or landline connections failed. The British military officers who lived in our apartment complex offered use of a generator in a pinch. We filled up the car with gas and spare tires—not that driving in a radioactive cloud would have been wise—and withdrew enough cash in case the banks shut.

On the fateful night, we went to Red Square with a group of friends—including, conveniently, the aforementioned members of Her Majesty's armed forces, who promised to whisk us out of the country if the situation got grave. We pocketed flashlights in case the streetlights failed and carried a few liters of champagne to douse fears. Then we held our breaths as Mother Russia counted down to midnight. The electricity stayed on. Corks popped. The Apocalypse failed to arrive, but we were primed just in case.

COMMUNICATION PLAN

A communication plan should list everyone to be contacted if you find yourself in an emergency. Such situations could be a tornado, an assault, falling on ice, an airline accident, or being arrested, pickpocketed, or teargassed. Contacts normally include one's significant other or next of kin, work associates, the children's school, local authorities, neighbors, animal and human doctors, and sometimes close friends and other relatives. List emails and phone numbers beside each name. You will provide all this information, and more, to a designated point person, or proxy, whose job it will be to reach out to everyone else when appropriate. Appointing one representative streamlines the communication process. Think of it as akin to an executor of a will, and make sure to seek the proxy's permission ahead of time to ensure that she or he is willing to assume such a weighty responsibility. You'll want to spare that person a surprise call that you're stranded in a wildfire, especially if it's a parent who frets unnecessarily about the most trifling matters. Let's just say that my late mother, may she rest in peace, was not the person to receive a distress call. She would automatically assume that I had one foot, if not two, in the grave. Better to select someone who will likely be

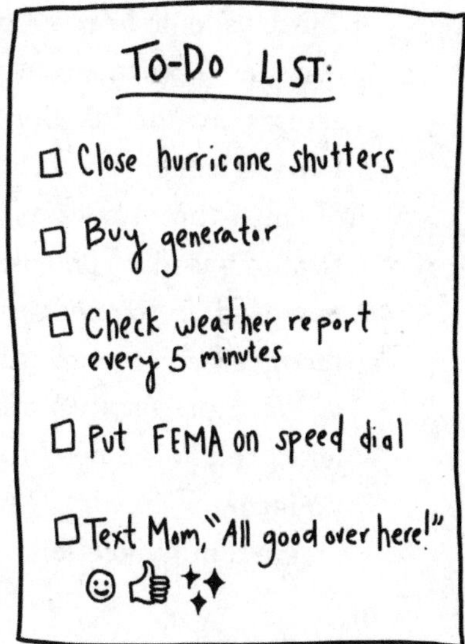

upset but who won't freeze in a panic when news arrives that you're hiding from an active shooter or are trapped in the cellar, or wherever, and who will coolly summon authorities to respond—the sort of person who doesn't blanche when a kid smashes a leg at a soccer game and the bone sticks out of his shin. This preternaturally composed individual must be someone you'd trust with your life, literally, because you will give this proxy a list not only of all your emergency contacts but also of the PIN codes and passwords to all your accounts and computers in the event that they are hacked or seized by scoundrels. The proxy will need access to all your financial files, and to know your blood type and passport number. The list should be in hard copy—that is, on paper—as it will contain so much sensitive information, and should not be sent as an email or Google Doc. Store it somewhere safe—like in a safe!

Once the proxy has agreed to take on the mammoth task of guarding your secrets, this sainted individual will make a plan to check in with you regularly should you be facing an emergency, such as sheltering in an attic during a hurricane or attending a protest that could turn violent. And you'll need to check in whenever the list needs updating.

The communication plan could look something like this:

Your full name:

Mobile phone and any other numbers:

Address:

Email:

Passwords and PINs for:

- Phone
- Computer
- Bank accounts

Names and info of important contacts such as the following:

- Partner
- Next of kin
- Employer
- Doctor
- Vet
- Lawyer
- Financial advisor (should you have one)

Your vital information:

- Date of birth
- Passport and Social Security numbers
- Blood type and any allergies or vital medications (e.g., insulin)
- Bank account numbers and passwords
- Other account numbers such as credit card, etc.
- Medical and property insurance

Itinerary in case of travel:

- Details of hotel
- Airline
- Vehicles
- Departure and arrival times
- Routes
- Reservation numbers

The communication plan should provide a general idea of how to proceed. (See page 275 for forms to use.) Now on to one of the most important lessons: dressing for dire events.

DRESS FOR SUCCESS

When I was based in Johannesburg, my boss, for reasons still unclear, bought me a burgundy bulletproof vest. It might have been a gender thing; I was the only woman on the team who covered civil wars and massacres on a regular basis. The guys, on the other hand, were awarded classic body armor that was the navy blue of a Brooks Brothers blazer. I've been all over the world, but to this day, I have never encountered anyone wearing a wine-colored flak jacket. Khaki, olive, camouflage, black, gray, and of course blue—yes. But crimson? Who wears crimson body armor in cross fire? No one! Granted, the color complemented my olive complexion, but I stood out as a target when rolling up to checkpoints.

As you can imagine, the eye-popping apparel created quite a stir among the trigger-nervous young men armed with AK-47 assault rifles who were guarding barricades. They were often stoned, as young men stationed at checkpoints tend to be, which undoubtedly made my jacket even more amusing. When I rolled up, they burst into hysterical guffaws and put down their guns in disbelief. The absurdity of the situation, I quickly learned, worked to my advantage—comedy is just what you need to leaven tension among nervous armed men high on weed and low on trust. You don't want them to think you're a menace, and a tiny woman wearing ridiculous attire does not appear threatening. And there's nothing like a weird outfit to jump-start conversation. (Consider wearing a red flak jacket to cocktail parties.) The gunslingers asked where I'd gotten it. *Why* I'd gotten it. Could they take a picture with me? They called their buddies over to get a look. Everyone chortled and handed around cigarettes and chatted with me about the weather. It occurred to me, as we bonded over fashion choices, that should my new BFFs decide to shoot me after all, the blood wouldn't leave a nasty stain. I wouldn't even have to wash it off—provided I survived of course. And there's more. The odd hue provided another unexpected protection. Security forces wore blue body armor, just like my male colleagues. So, the male reporters were often mistakenly shot at in cross fire. But no one shot at *moi*.

While random, the choice of the red garment taught me a powerful lesson. Details such as fabric and cultural appropriateness go a long way toward conserving life. Dressing properly is a critical component to success, success being safety.

You're probably wondering, What does this have to do with me? I don't plan to go to a war zone, and I don't like the color red.

Stay with me. The same outfitting principle applies to protest rallies, wildfires, hurricanes, insects, and sudden swings in weather in the wilderness. Natural disasters are on the rise, and each year, backpackers die from falls and exposure. Zika-infected mosquitoes can bite through thin socks. And a heeled sandal can trip you up in a shopping crush. Lest this seem a frivolous concern, consider the crucial role cloth and style have played throughout history (beyond shopping at Saks, that is). Hannibal lost an estimated fourteen thousand men on his 218 BC march across the Alps partly because they wore flimsy garments and footwear in the snow. In those days, no one had Gore-Tex boots, so Hannibal's men froze to death or plunged off precipices for lack of traction. You could, too, if you went on a protest march or trekked without the right boots.

The following are the essentials of my safety wardrobe:

Ode to the Ecco Boot

Speaking of footwear, if the shoe fits, don't necessarily wear it. Ditch the sneakers. They don't provide sufficient ankle support. Instead, head to the nearest camping supply store and intone, "Ecco." Adherents of such outdoors establishments have no doubt come across this comfy and lightweight Gore-Tex wonder. It's resilient and, being Danish, ensures Scandinavian flair as you sprint to safety. If you can't find Eccos that fit or you don't like this season's style, any lightweight waterproof hiking boot will do. You won't regret it. I have never met a climate my Eccos didn't thrive in. If I were a religious person, I would bow down and pray to this shoe. I have worn mine on glaciers and in the Congo jungle. I have trekked with them in Nepal. They've stomped on centipedes in Kenya. And they've never failed in their sturdy grip. Over thirty years of constant wear, I have replaced mine only once because they last forever, or almost forever; this saves a lot of money. In the intervening years, I replaced the insoles when they began to stink. I abuse my shoes, and these have always withstood the challenge. Unlike friends, the Ecco is always forgiving and reliable.

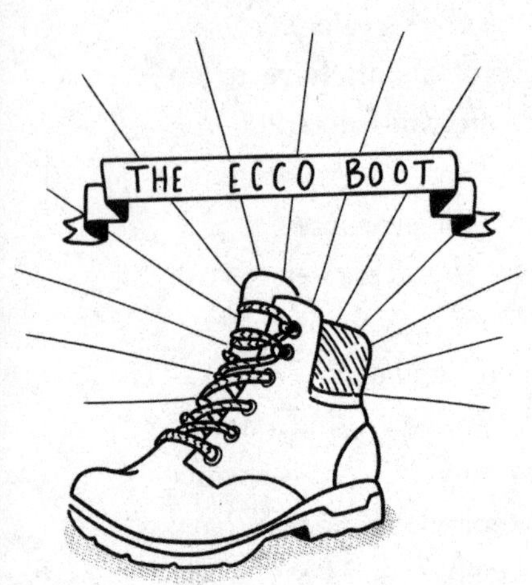

Cross-body Bag

This wildly ergonomic bag that slings over the chest is more comfortable and secure than a backpack. Anyone can grab a backpack while it's on your back and slice it with a knife. Not the over-the-shoulder bag, which is also easy to run with and is better for one's posture. Its many compartments allow one to distribute and reach for essentials like phones and lipstick with ease. It can hold nearly as much as a day pack and is waterproof. I favor the Victoronix mainly because I found one on sale for $10, but the internet offers plenty of other models to choose from. Don't report to field duty without it!

Climate Extremes

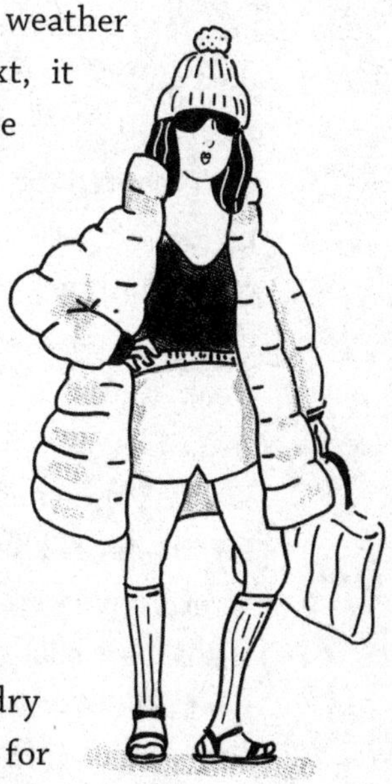

Each year, hikers and mountaineers suffer injuries or even death from falling ice or harsh cold. The biggest challenge for me when researching my book about mountains and conflict, which took me to eight ranges around the world, was not encountering guerrilla groups but dressing for dramatic swings in temperature. One moment, the weather broiled at seventy-five degrees; the next, it snowed. The way the climate is going these days, such extremes are becoming the new normal all over the place. Just the other day, when I was in Colorado, the temperature swung a record seventy degrees over a twenty-four-hour period. Seventy degrees! For that we should all be shopping at REI, even for everyday wear. In order to dress for such eventualities, I have layers on hand whatever the forecast. If I'm going to a cold climate, merino wool sweaters and long underwear, which dry quickly and are thin but warm, are added for extra warmth on top of the usual staples. Socks should be made of fabric that wicks away perspiration. I find lightweight hiking socks made of wool versatile for a variety of climates, and they serve as a fine barrier against biting insects. Utility aside, it's also more economical to dress in layers than to have distinct sets of clothing for every season. These days, outdoors brands like Patagonia make outer and undergarments that can be worn with a suit to the office. As well as climatic emergencies, they do double duty for political demonstrations and travel.

Eyeglasses versus Surgery

Unsecured eyeglasses can fall off when you're running, and there is nothing more frightening than having them ripped off your face when you're being interrogated, or facing down a tornado when you can't see because your specs got blown off. Yet contact lenses are unwise during a teargassing or a dust storm. So, after losing myriad pairs of glasses and contracting infections from dirt and other stuff flying into my eyes, I opted for laser surgery on my corneas. I was haunted by the experience of a colleague in Russia who jumped onto a military patrol without his Bausch & Lomb case. He thought it was a day trip, but the operation lasted nearly a week, and after wearing the same pair of contacts the entire time, he emerged with scratched corneas and pink eye. Various branches of the American military offer the surgery for myopic soldiers precisely for that reason. With the photorefractive keratectomy option, otherwise known as PRK, the doctor slices the outside of the cornea before applying the laser to reshape it. In contrast, the more sophisticated Lasik procedure creates a flap of tissue and then goes in with the laser. The flip side to both these surgeries is that some people suffer from side effects such as dry eye and halos around lights, so do a risk assessment to judge whether going without glasses is worth it. It was for me. Aside from coping with tear gas better, I can finally see the clock when I'm in a swimming pool.

Ready-to-Go Bag

As a foreign correspondent, I had to be prepared for unforeseen events that could erupt at any given moment. A car bomb might go off down the road, or I'd have to rush to the airport to cover a coup two countries away. Maybe a bus crashed nearby, or someone invited me to a party! That meant always keeping a packed bag at my desk or in the car's trunk, with a variety of outfits for any occasion. While the ordinary American is unlikely to be called to cover a revolution, you might suddenly find yourself stranded by any manner of inclement weather. That's where the ready-to-go bag comes in. I still keep one by my desk. Mine contains toiletries and a change of clothes for two weeks, a medical kit, rain gear, spare batteries, and cables—all neatly tucked away. The carrier serves two purposes. One, I don't have to rush to pack. Two, I save the energy I would have wasted debating what to wear, a perennial misery that torments me. To keep things simple, I choose three outfits, all in black (to hide dirt), hand-washable, and quick drying for rinsing in a sink each night. The color coordination means I can interchange the shirts and trousers. (It also increases the chic quotient considerably.) I also keep the bag packed for ordinary travel. (More on that in the next chapter.) Every garment hangs below thigh level, so as not to offend people in conservative cultures and, now, later in life, to hide menopausal bulges. (Why do you think Eileen Fisher makes money? She's cornered the tunic market among women of a certain age.) Jeans don't join the mix. They are made of heavy fabric, so they take forever to dry. And light blue shows dirt. I also set aside special travel shoes—the aforementioned running boots and a fancier pair with heels, but not so delicate that they can get stuck in between cobblestones or in mud.

Condoms

I know what you're thinking, but correspondents of all genders keep rubbers around, and not just to ward off semen and STDs. Condoms make great containers for water and can keep supplies (e.g., blister bandages) dry. Survivalists use them as gloves and tourniquets and to start fires. And if you don't have a way to defend yourself, you can fill them with water and hurl them at an attacker. Never travel without 'em!

Medical Kit

Don't ride out a freak storm without a medical kit. After all, you won't be able to pop out to a Rite Aid for supplies. The first tier of the kit should contain two weeks' worth of supplies of over-the-counter essentials. These include burn cream, bandages, splints, aspirin or Tylenol, ibuprofen, antibacterial cream, antihistamines, chewable Pepto-Bismol, stronger antidiarrhea meds like Imodium, and hydrocortisone cream.

The second tier consists of more alarming supplies; consult chapter 4 ("Just Plug It—Emergency First Aid") for more details. These should include a card with blood type and any chronic conditions (e.g., diabetes); water purification pills; rehydration tablets; rolls of gauze (to stick inside someone's pelvic cavity or elsewhere); bandaging material, including pressurized ACE wraps, safety pins, and shears or scissors; a CPR mask; latex gloves; goggles (in case contaminated blood sprays in your face); syringes; and tourniquets. (A warning about the last item: Make sure you know how to use a tourniquet properly. This is very serious. You don't want someone to have a limb amputated because you tied the tourniquet too tight or in the wrong place.)

The third tier comprises medications that require a prescription, including antibiotics for a wide range of ailments and, if relevant, an inhaler, EpiPen, Diflucan (generic name: fluconazole) for yeast infections, and insulin.

Finally, keep handy emergency snacks such as trail mix and dried fruit. I count these as medical essentials. When you're hungry you can't think straight, which can have fatal implications.

Be Safe with a Safe

Make copies of every important document, such as your passport, other identification, driver's license, birth certificate, and medical and financial files and put them in a secure place, like a fireproof safe. My husband and I installed one at our place in New York, to save us worrying about theft or loss. We got into the habit years earlier, when we lived in Johannesburg, the land of the frequent house break-in. The practice also offers peace of mind in the event of natural catastrophes. The safe has a greater chance of surviving than the house itself.

TALKING TO KIDS ABOUT SCARY EVENTS

One of the greatest challenges parents encounter in this unsettled world is keeping their kids calm in the face of an emergency. We want them to feel secure yet prepared in case true disaster strikes.

The adults should sit down and have a conversation about perceived and real threats. Generally, teens get it and will welcome tools that make them feel more in control. Some young kids are easily spooked, and we don't want to destroy their last shred of safety. Make it less scary by involving them in the preparations. Unlike teenagers, the younger ones love important jobs. Take them along to the hardware store to buy the supplies, and let them pick out their own special flashlight. Delegate tasks to them, such as packing their favorite toys and games. Enlist them to check the weather report with you every day. At the very least, they'll be able to alert the family when you need to bring along an umbrella.

As for school shootings, I've been struck by how many of the high school students I've met have done drills in their schools, such as hiding quietly in a closet, and then emerged feeling deeply upset by the experience. Clearly, drills for disasters like earthquakes and tornadoes are less upsetting because they are for natural acts. A storm doesn't target you, and generally kids don't get rattled by such exercises. School shootings are another matter. If such drills cause your child apprehension, talk to the school about the messaging in order to ensure that everyone is on the same page and not causing undue alarm. In fact, I suggest talking to the school ahead of time to find out what practices it follows.

An exercise should provide a sense of agency while not triggering acute anxiety, especially for children under the age of twelve. Many students today are already conditioned to know a shooting may occur. One shouldn't increase their fears with hyperrealistic scenarios involving fake blood and adults pretending to shoot students.

Take the case of the 2018 massacre at Marjory Stoneman Douglas High School in Parkland, Florida. One of the survivors, Ryan Deitsch, told me about an active shooter drill years earlier when he was in the fifth grade that troubled him and other classmates greatly. It didn't necessarily prepare him for the real event that occurred years later. As he tells it, the ten-year-olds were directed to hide in a bathroom without much contact with their teacher. They received no warning ahead of time and huddled claustrophobically, shoulder to shoulder, for what seemed like a couple of hours. That's not the best practice. Kids shouldn't fear that they might die, and they generally don't take to being told to consider survival right before a math test. As long as they are familiar with what to do, they will get through a real-life situation. Having a plan, such as knowing where the exits are and to remain quiet, is more constructive for young people than actively simulating a terrifying experience. Moreover, appropriate training should be done for the teachers and staff so that they can handle such an emotionally charged experience. (The Resources section details the best practices recommended by leading school security and child development experts.)

I think back to kindergarten, when drills for nuclear attack were done in a non-alarmist manner. The year was 1963, the height of Cold War hysteria. Like many public schools, my own, PS 32, held duck-and-cover exercises. The teacher would call out, "Now!" and we kids would drop under our wooden desks and curl into human balls. (Never mind that hiding under a desk wouldn't really protect you from an atomic bomb.) The teacher smartly didn't mention anything about possible obliteration. On the contrary, she made the exercise seem mundane, if pointless. I had no idea that she worried about Russian strikes. I didn't even know the Russians had bombs, or what those bombs did. I knew they had Matryoshka nesting dolls because my grandmother had brought me one from Moscow. The teacher was so (seemingly) matter-of-fact during the drills that the only thing that alarmed me was a stain on the carpet. A kid named Clifford had vomited there earlier, and I went into contortions to avoid the puke mark. We practiced ducking and rolling so many times, with me deftly avoiding Clifford's stain, that the routine became rote. It's so ingrained in my muscle memory that I could do it today with the right prompt, fifty-five years later.

Meanwhile, back at home—in the two-family detached brick house that looked like all the neighbors'—my parents stocked the basement closet with nonperishable food. Supplies included biscuits that tasted like chalk, Campbell's tomato soup, and enough cans of tuna to last six months and give you so much mercury that you'd be drooling at the mouth and going a bit loony. But my parents weren't thinking about contaminated tuna then. This was about threats that didn't fit in a can. My folks also stashed dried milk and, as a special treat, plastic jars of marshmallow creme. We spread this Marshmallow Fluff, as the popular sugary concoction was called, on white Wonder Bread with peanut butter. The ensuing "Fluffernutter" sandwich looked like cat diarrhea and, from a health perspective, should have been the last thing a human ate in a toxic, radioactive environment, but it was all the rage among East Coast schoolchildren. (See Resources.) But I digress. One might argue that my family's brimming cellar pantry was stocked for convenience as well as emergency. Being cheap, a dominant gene in my family, we saved money by buying in bulk with coupons, of which my parents were avid collectors. When asked about why he had accumulated so much stuff, my dad didn't say anything about miserly tendencies. (This was pre-Costco.) Rather, the piles of tin cans were there "just in case," although in case of *what* he never revealed.

The point I'm making here is that the adults around me were so low-key about the potential of annihilation that I wasn't a bit alarmed. I think back to those preparations with memories as sweet as that Marshmallow Fluff. We went through the drop-and-roll motions at school, counting the minutes until we could go out to play on the slides and munch on Fluffernutters during recess. That's the way it should be—preparations that become automatic but not panic inducing. Like fire drills.

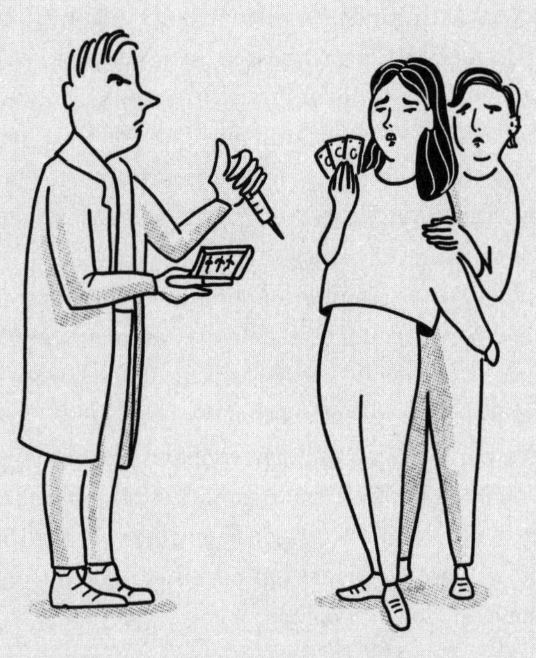

Chapter 3

BRING IT ON—TRAVEL

A few years back, I flew into an African country with a British magazine writer who was new to the region. Unbeknownst to my travel companion, a lot of countries outside Europe require proof of vaccination against dangerous diseases. With their collapsed health services and open sewers, impoverished countries can be breeding grounds for infections, epidemics, and bacteria. This particular nation was notorious for every illness for which one should get vaccinated—measles, cholera, mumps, yellow fever, typhoid, hepatitis of all letters, typhus, meningitis, tuberculosis, encephalitis, polio, rabies, rubella, diphtheria, tetanus, whooping cough, chickenpox, HIV, and at least one flu case. As we approached the immigration desk at the airport, a pleasant man in a white coat asked to see our vaccination stamps for yellow fever. Anyone who entered the country had to be inoculated, he explained. The British journalist fumbled in her bag, but alas, the international health booklet was back at the house.

She had gotten the vaccination, but didn't have the required evidence. "Not to worry," White Coat said. "We can give you the shot right here." He then pulled out an enormous syringe that appeared rusted (or perhaps was merely covered in dried blood from the previous passenger). The British woman trembled. All blood drained from her face. She frantically searched her bag again. Nothing. "You can pay a fine," the gentleman suggested, winking repeatedly, in case she didn't get his drift. She pulled out a fistful of twenty-dollar bills, far more than the going bribery rate, and the sinister needle returned to its box.

This should serve as a cautionary tale: Do a checklist before you go anywhere. There are so many things to consider besides the risk of being jabbed with a potentially fatal syringe. Before I take a trip, I ponder the following about my destination: any known conflicts, the color of the taxis, dangerous animals, inclement weather, the local equivalent of 911, sartorial no-nos, local customs, contact number for the U.S. consulate, the local type of electrical outlets and voltage, and a safe hotel.

Also ask:

What special gear should I pack?

Whom do I stay in touch with while traveling?

Does my phone have international roaming? (If not, get it in advance.)

What affairs should I put in order before leaving?

Do I need to translate important documents into the local language?

How might I be perceived by potentially hostile people, such as governments or waiters?

Let's look at these considerations in more detail.

BEFORE YOU GO

Shots (Not from Guns)

The immunization booklet piles up plaudits among foreign correspondents for reasons I've just made clear. This handy item has entries for all the recommended or required shots, to help you keep track of when you got inoculated and how long the vaccination will last. (I also recommend keeping up to date with yearly flu shots.) When you're jabbed, the doctor or medical center provides a dated stamp on the relevant page. Many doctors do not know what vaccines are needed for a particular country, so you should make it a point to check the websites for the Centers for Disease Control and Prevention and the World Health Organization. (See Resources.) I keep my immunization booklet up to date and never fail to pack it.

Pre-trip Jitters

I've traveled more than a million miles over my four-decade journalism career. That works out to about twenty-five thousand miles a year. You'd think that the process would be a breeze by now. Not so! I get the heebie-jeebies before nearly every trip, especially when it's for pleasure. Seriously. I have trouble sleeping, and stress over what catastrophe might occur (although I do, admittedly, get excited about my frequent-flyer status). I fret about theft, sickness, and that my family won't miss me. What if I'm detained upon arrival?

What if I lose my cell phone in the terminal? What if the airline overbooked and I miss my appointments the next day? What if we crash? I check and recheck that my MacBook Air is powered up. I check and recheck that my passport is still valid, even though I renewed it only a year ago. I worry about getting to the airport on time. What if there's an earthquake and the road splits in half and then the taxi gets rear-ended and the driver is pulled over for hitting a motorcyclist and then a thief rides up and robs us? You know, likely scenarios for missing flights. I compensate by leaving extra early, and I mean ludicrously extra early, like three hours, to face all these unlikely scenarios. It's a source of pride for me that during my one million miles of travel, I have never missed a flight. It's a source of intense irritation for everyone else around me. My family groans every time we go on holiday because I try to force them to leave so much in advance that we sit in the airport lounge longer than the actual flight to Amsterdam from New York.

Yet harnessing this edginess to my advantage and listening to those concerns actually helps me identify potential pitfalls. Visualizing the worst-case scenario makes me realize that so many of my anxieties, about being cut off from the familiar or losing things, are overblown. By contemplating extreme situations, I go through a checklist of how to avoid them or deal with them. So, by the time I get on the plane, I'm halfway to Zen.

In order to make travel even less stressful, for myself as well as for the people I torment, my suitcase (a carry-on, of course) remains packed all the time and stored in a closet. Such preparations provide me one less thing to worry about. This means the tiny toiletries and collapsible umbrella remain in the bag even after I return home. So does the passport and copies thereof, vaccination card, earphones (to avoid paying seven dollars onboard for crappy ones that don't work), plug adapters, and spare batteries, pens, and reading glasses. (Lasik resolved only the myopia.) As soon as I book a flight or hotel, a printed copy of the reservation goes into the carry-on. (Another common fear: I won't be able to scan the ticket at the check-in desk.) I have a limited number of travel outfits per climate, to avoid vacillating over choices. Also, I quickly replace items that expire or run out so that the bag remains filled.

Wills and Things

Foreign correspondents have a sloppy habit of leaving financial affairs in a mess. I suspect people of most professions do as well. This oversight becomes problematic if they get killed. Loved ones then don't know where to find important documents, like wills. It's bad enough that your family is grieving (assuming they miss you). Don't make it worse by leaving zero instructions for distributing your wealth. One colleague always asks employees the sobering question "Have you made arrangements to repatriate your body?" While that's probably going too far for a Christmas break in Miami, making arrangements for someone to find your legal documents in case of an untimely demise might not be. Such documents include powers of attorney, living wills, your lawyer's contact details, and so on. Have you appointed an executor? This is where you hark back to the proxy in chapter 1, the friend, relative, or colleague who knows where to locate all files, passwords, loved ones, and employers in case of an emergency. Think of it as akin to carrying an umbrella (the non-flimsy kind) so that it doesn't rain. You know, Murphy's Law. If you have the umbrella, it won't rain.

Choosing the Right Hotel

I love my work, but not when I travel solo. Unfortunately, I have to travel solo much of the time. Even though the catcalls and come-ons have lessened with age—viva menopause!—I often feel like I stick out like a llama when I check into a hotel alone in many countries. In order to make sure I'm not staying in the middle of a prostitution district, or on the square where rioters habitually run amok, I assiduously research the safest hotels and neighborhoods to base myself in, as well as taxi companies whose drivers don't have a reputation for robbing or raping customers. The U.S. State Department offers a safety checklist for before you go, including cultural considerations if you're LGBTQ or of a particular faith. I also check news reports, trawl online sites like Lonely Planet and TripAdvisor, and ask acquaintances and Facebook friends for referrals.

I learned this lesson all too well during an assignment to Dagestan, a Muslim republic of Russia undergoing an extended rebellion. I made the mistake of staying at a hotel with a bar. Normally, a stiff whisky would be desirable after a day of interviewing torture victims, and my coworker made a booking at a hotel with a twenty-four-hour drinking supply. (I'm not referring to potable water.) However, she didn't realize that Islamic extremists were bombing establishments that sold alcohol. The reservation could have been a fatal mistake. Luckily the militants targeted liquor stores during our stay. We had dodged a bullet or, rather, a pipe bomb. And we made good use of the bar once we learned this.

We all have a bottom line for the standards we seek in travel, and security is mine. I'm willing to pay more for a guard in the lobby and a safe to lock up valuables. I'll opt for a centrally located hotel chain over an Airbnb any day or night. I began to appreciate the virtues of a reputable hotel when I worked for Reuters a few decades ago. In the halcyon days of this multinational corporation, bosses expected staff to stay at the best digs in town. Five-star lodging helped forge professional contacts, so the logic went. At first, I suspected that the honchos simply preferred minibars stocked with Chivas rather than some mundane Scotch. Who wouldn't? But with time, I recognized the added wisdom of not skimping on accommodation. Should a crisis descend, a good hotel has backup generators and reliable communications. It has enormous freezers to store food. When I stayed in the Intercontinental in Kinshasa, the manager was able to serve fresh croissants every morning during an uprising. What's more, he offered the roof to any embassy that wanted to land helicopters to evacuate guests. No one took him up on that offer, but I found the gesture classy. You don't get that kind of service with Airbnb.

Besides helipads, I consider amenities a safety issue, too. My worst-case scenario is that I can't get a Caesar salad after curfew or there's no treadmill to work off stress. After a rough day of sightseeing or inhaling tear gas, this tired traveler desires 24/7 room service. Oh, and excellent Wi-Fi so that I can check emails. I make better decisions when rested and well fed. Also, I prefer hotels that offer a front desk that can call a reliable taxi and provide advice on where to change money and find a doctor if necessary. As a solo traveler, I'm a big fan of hotel lobby restaurants and bars that cater to businesspeople. These sterile environs are more conducive to your being left alone, and they save you from having to go out solo at night. Staff are more likely to intervene if an annoying customer sends drinks to your table or, worse, barges in to join you. Aside from the aforementioned attributes, I also like a stuff-yourself breakfast that fuels me through the day. Hotels lose money when Matloff heads to the buffet. I may look small, but I always pack in a giant early chow, especially when it's included in the room rate.

SPOTLIGHT ON AIRBNB

If you do choose Airbnb, avoid nighttime arrival when traveling solo. If a red-eye flight is your only option, consider checking into a chain hotel at the airport the night you land, before moving to the Airbnb when light breaks.

Airbnb claims it screens international hosts against terrorism and sanctions watch lists and conducts background checks for hosts in the United States. It will also provide smoke detectors if requested. But there's no guarantee your host will ask for one, or won't be a first-time rapist or thief. To minimize the risk of assault, stay in places that have an impressive bouquet of excellent reviews over a long period, especially ones written by single women and families. Message reviewers privately through the site's internal mail system to glean more information about the host. Rent the entire apartment and avoid shares. If traveling alone, stay with a female host or a couple. Share your details with contacts back home. Airbnb offers a safety hotline if you get into trouble, but don't expect them to call the cavalry to get you out.

THE LIFE-CHANGING MAGIC OF CARRY-ON LUGGAGE

Here's Matloff rule number one: Only bring what you can run with. This skill has gained serious relevancy as airlines increasingly charge for even one check-in bag. It also makes it easier (read: safer) in case you have to rush off a plane that has caught fire. I got into this habit while traveling to places where I actually had to sprint with my baggage, due to shelling or because I had overslept and risked missing the plane. I weigh less than a hundred pounds, so I can't run with much. I also like to keep my belongings on my person; I've lost too many bags in transit in countries where the airport staff steal or slit passengers' luggage. It didn't get "misdirected." Someone actually made off with it. (A solution is slash-proof luggage, of course.)

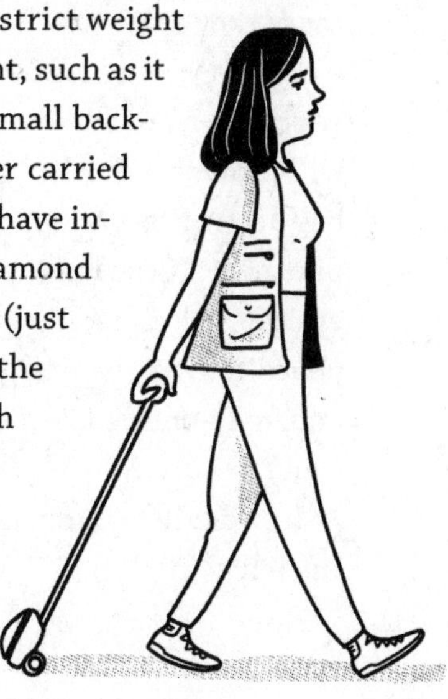

Another reason I travel light: I often flew on helicopters or eight-seat planes that lacked the cargo space of proper commercial jets. Light aircraft have strict weight limits, and the storage compartment, such as it is, is large enough to stash only a small backpack or assault rifle. (Not that I ever carried the latter, but my fellow passengers have included mercenaries, soldiers, and diamond smugglers.) My one allotted duffel (just one) went into a tiny section behind the last seat of the plane, or would perch on my lap. (Seat belt requirements tend to be loose on mercenary planes.) Once, in Mali, I was able to sneak aboard a second bag, but then another passenger brought on a live goat. The animal took up most of the luggage space and looked ready to crap on the bags piled around it. I hoped that the goat would have second thoughts about joining us and would get off the plane, but then the pilot firmly tied its rope to the last seat and began looking for something to throw off the plane in its place. He chose my shoulder bag containing a couple of changes of dirty clothes, several fat paperbacks, and my Bausch & Lomb contact solution. I suddenly had a transformational epiphany, no doubt what Marie Kondo experienced the first time she tidied a closet. A mammoth weight left my soul along with that bag. My gosh. I didn't need all that stuff! I felt liberated! Ever since that enlightening moment, traveling ultra-light has been my creed, much to the relief of my long-suffering husband, who used to get stuck carrying my suitcases. (The man is a saint.) Whether on a business trip or vacation, I channel my inner KonMari and pack only the bare essentials, although less because they spark joy than because I actually *need* them.

Before we discuss what to pack in the carry-on, consider your actions in a true emergency. An aisle seat near an exit will provide a quicker getaway. Keep your valuables in the bag by your feet as opposed to the one in the overhead compartment. If you have to evacuate quickly, you won't hold up everyone else's escape fumbling to get a bag down. This happened during the emergency landing of an Aeroflot plane, and forty-one people died unable to get out in time. Seconds count.

In order to maximize space, my carry-on luggage contains the following:

Old Clothes

I often travel with worn-out T-shirts and socks to sleep or exercise in, which I then junk at the end of the trip. There's nothing like flying home with less than you started with, and my inner Marie Kondo knows to get rid of things that don't spark joy. I also wash as much clothing as I can in the bathroom sink and then hang it up to dry. Hotel shampoo and shower gel are great stand-ins for laundry detergent and are normally gentle enough for delicates. Hand-washing saves on laundry bills or having to pack too many outfits. For those new to hand-washing: Check the labels to ensure the clothes are not "dry clean only." If you get the all-clear, fill the basin with cold water or whatever water temperature the label recommends. Add shampoo or soap, let sit for five minutes, and then rinse and wring until the suds disappear. Hang up to dry.

Rain Gear

You just never know about the weather these days. So, bring a collapsible umbrella and a waterproof poncho—even in dry climates because, well, you never know what climate change will bring. True to its collapsible name, the umbrella will get bent out of shape in light wind, so you won't have to lug it home at the end of the trip.

Small Packs of Toilet Paper

Self-explanatory. You never know.

Headlamp Flashlight

These lights surpass any other form of travel illumination, including the iPhone. Strapped on the forehead, they free up the hands when you're stumbling from the poolside bar to your hotel room, or typing outside in the dark, or trying to find your room key. They're great for night hikes. Various options exist, including triple-A-battery-powered, mini LED, and USB-rechargeable.

Flip-Flops

These are de rigueur for everything from poolsides to filthy latrines. Those flat paper sandals they give you at nice hotels rarely fit properly, and they don't offer traction on slippery surfaces.

Camping Towel

Quick-drying camping towels make sense if you don't like the fiber count of the hotel towels or you have a thing about using other people's bath accessories in the Airbnb.

Cotton Sheet

The same principle applies to the cotton sheet as to the camping towel, but this one serves more purposes. I picked up the practice of bringing along my own cotton sheets in Mozambique, where women wrap them around their waists in lieu of skirts and sling babies in them on their backs. I wind mine around me on the way to the hotel pool, and then use it as a germ barrier if the pillow stinks of the previous guests. These sheets make great liners for sleeping bags and, being quick-drying, can double as towels. I also string them up for privacy during al fresco toileting when I'm surrounded by men on military bases or camping trips, and discreetly change my underwear underneath them. They fold into nothing.

Photocopies

Make copies of every important document, such as reservations, passport, identification, driver's license, and credit card hotline. Store one in the hotel safe and keep another on your person. If the police demand your passport, hand over the photocopy and politely tell them to call the embassy if they have an issue with that. (Also, keep the telephone number and address of the consulate handy in case of trouble.) You have to show the actual passport to exchange money at banks, but try not to let it fall into the hands of men with guns, especially in countries renowned for corruption.

Burner Phones

These disposable throwaways look like flip phones from the days of old, before people had Instagram or had heard of cat videos. Burners are cheaper and harder to track than smartphones, which makes me think burners are actually more intelligent than smartphones. I bought one of these babies for about twenty dollars in Mexico, and simply get a local SIM card when in other countries. Foreign correspondents who travel frequently tape their various SIM cards to the phone, for easy access in case they're suddenly summoned to fly to Sierra Leone or Tashkent. They leave the smartphone in the hotel safe and then tool around town with the burner. That way, it won't have any sensitive info on it in case of its theft or seizure.

Small Electronics

A no-brainer. Journalists carry lots of gear that can be stolen or confiscated, so less is more—as long as it doesn't sacrifice quality. I worship cameras I can sneak into my pocket.

I kneel to the Kindle god. As a journalist, I often find myself stuck waiting for hours, if not days or, in some cases, weeks, for a flight or a lift. That's something that travelers on Thanksgiving weekend can relate to, no doubt. Reading matter keeps me as sane as I can be. I wrote my first book, all 318 pages, sitting in airports waiting for delayed helicopters and cargo planes. One time, in Timbuktu, I got bumped off the once-weekly flight because a Mali government official wanted my seat. I had to wait three days to arrange a jeep to take me to a barge down the Niger River and then onward by road to the nation's capital, Bamako. By the end of the journey, I had finished *War and Peace* and made headway in *Remembrance of Things Past*. Nowadays, I always make sure the Kindle is powered up before I depart, in case the power source blows during a hurricane or other calamity. The reading light can double as a flashlight.

The same goes for laptops: Light is might. And just as important as weight is protecting personal information contained on the computer. What with hacking these days, I'm paranoid that someone will get ahold of my sensitive information. Potential adversaries range from competitive colleagues and snooping governments to my own kid. So, I travel with a "dummy" laptop. During my last trip to Russia, I used a three-hundred-dollar notebook with nothing of import on it. Anyone who searched it—which was no doubt the intelligence goons sitting 24/7 outside my hotel room—found boring messages about my son's soccer schedule. Just to make life hard for them, I used a special email account set up exclusively for the trip, one that had no links to anything in my past. Then I stored the dummy laptop under my dirtiest clothes so any snoop would have to rifle through the disgusting heap to get to the electronics. I actually felt sort of sorry for the guys (but not so sorry that I wouldn't do it again).

Correct Plugs

You'd be amazed at how many hardened pros show up on foreign assignments with the wrong electrical plug. They forget to check ahead of time if the destination country uses 110 or 120 voltage, or a two-peg plug versus a three. But then, who hasn't at some point tried to force a square peg into a round hole? Or plug in a 110-voltage laptop without a 220 adapter? That will burn out the equipment. The opposite, plugging a 220 into a 110, will fail to power up the device. No good can come of such mishaps for correspondents. Our work relies on charged cell phones, laptops, cameras, voice recorders, video cameras, satellite telephones, and hair dryers. One of my cohorts missed a giant story while running around in search of an adapter during the 1997 rebellion in Zaire. By the time he found one, the rebels had seized control and renamed the country the Democratic Republic of Congo. We renamed his career: Over. Such mishaps can ruin a beach sojourn, too. Who wants to waste valuable snorkel time driving to electronics stores in search of an adapter? No one. An easy solution beckons: the world plug, sold at chain drugstores and the bigger airports. Up to a point, however. Last I counted, our planet boasts about fifteen different kinds of plugs, and only the most common varieties are included in the world plug.

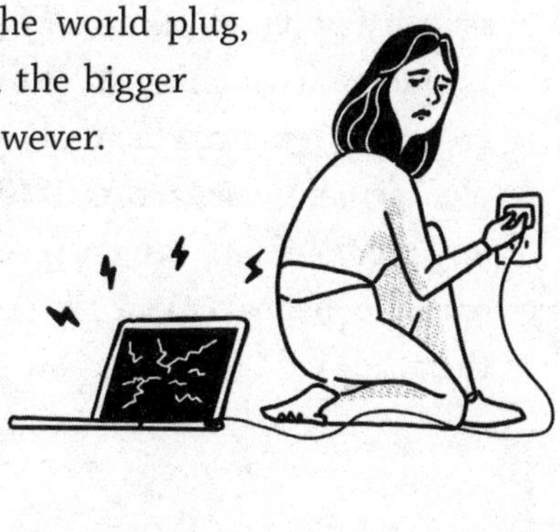

My super-duper model, which I bought in the Warsaw airport, has only seven. To make life further difficult, some countries use both up-to-date sockets and older variants that haven't been replaced. To be safe, check the world plug guide of the International Electrotechnical Commission—yes, there is such a thing—for a full list of who uses what where. (See Resources.)

Toiletries

I rely on the soap/shampoo/conditioner/lotion/gel combos provided in hotel bathrooms. You can lift spares for your next trip from the housekeeping cart in the hall. The quality often sucks, but hair can stand a couple days of sulfate washes without falling out. Most important, these tiny bottles don't take up much room in the suitcase, which gets us back to the carry-on safety issue. Other amenities, like razors or toothpaste, can usually be obtained by calling down to reception. For more refined beauty items like cosmetics and perfume, check out Sephora's travel products. Some are so small you can barely see them. I recently scored a lipstick about the size of a grape; the thing weighs maybe an ounce. The one item missing from my toiletry bag is a set of plastic tweezers that can go through the metal detectors at airport security. I don't think anyone makes them, and I often think I could get rich doing so. While this Holy Grail of personal grooming remains elusive, I make sure my eyebrows are well plucked before departing. If they grow back while I'm traveling, I hide behind sunglasses—or scrape the pesky hairs off with the disposal razor provided by hotel housekeeping and then hide behind sunglasses. Ah, the price of beauty.

DRESS FOR SUCCESS

Weighing ninety-nine pounds and having sickly pale skin and hair that defies combs, I stick out in any environment other than an old age home, even if I'm not wearing a red flak jacket. For that reason, I pay extraordinary attention to being minimally conspicuous when traveling overseas. I don't want to call attention to myself as a potential hostage, or simply an ugly American. Being unobtrusive leads to lower taxi fares, polite treatment at restaurants, and fewer conversations about American politics. You're also less likely to be pickpocketed.

Several colleagues of mine cover their blond hair with caps in order to merge into crowds in places like Mexico, even while on vacation. Sometimes wearing the local garb makes you look like you're about to trick-or-treat. Try as I may, I never managed to drape a sari without it unraveling at inopportune moments, and I trip in burqas. (It's difficult to see through the mesh over the eyes.) If you can't pull off the look convincingly, then opt for conservative Western dress. And it goes without saying that you shouldn't wear shorts or go sleeveless if the locals don't. Ultimately, the way you carry yourself will determine your success.

One of my favorite go-to items is a diaphanous black scarf that a friend gifted to me in Chechnya. It's appropriate for houses of worship in Islamic countries, where female heads should be covered, and it's a godsend on bad hair days anywhere else. I wrap it around my greasy locks if I don't have an opportunity to shampoo. It's light enough for the 120-degree weather that will soon be the norm, and can double as a festive wrap at colder fêtes.

I always pack a lightweight black dress that can serve as both party attire and a cover-up when I'm heading to the hotel pool. One that reaches the ankles is ideal for situations where exposed flesh can prompt unwanted grabs or even a flogging. I favor stretchy items that are hand-washable and can be rolled up to the size of a tennis ball. (This saves suitcase room for the bulky bulletproof vest or other clothes.) The operational term for all items is *quick dry*, as garments washed every night shouldn't be damp or mildewed the next morning.

One caveat for the color scheme: Black's an unwise choice if you travel to a place where only widows or paramilitaries wear it. After all, you don't want to look like you're coming from a funeral or causing someone else's.

STAYING SAFE WHILE YOU'RE THERE

When possible while I'm abroad, I'll contact anyone I might know in town for advice or even to meet for a meal. I also ask acquaintances for introductions to locals. It doesn't hurt to know someone in your destination country in case a crisis unfolds. I derive immense peace of mind from the communication plan mentioned in chapter 1, which you have, of course, committed to memory. I regularly check in with my husband, who has a copy of my itinerary and knows my daily plan. If you're staying in a hotel, ask staff about the protocols for emergencies (another advantage over an Airbnb), such as power outages, fires, and storms. Stay abreast of news updates if one of these occurs. I also suggest registering in the

State Department's Smart Traveler Enrollment Program, which issues security alerts and contacts you in case of an emergency situation. It will also let you know about events at embassies, such as Fourth of July celebrations, if you're in the market for free food.

Commonsense Safety

I'm sure you know not to do this, but I'll say it anyway. Don't walk around with your face in your phone. Walking with your eyes down can invite muggers or cause you to step into oncoming traffic. Also, always carry on your person the address and phone number of the hotel in case you get lost. However, when going out to eat solo, it's wise to bury your face in a magazine or your Kindle, and put on your best resting bitch face so that you look unapproachable. If you just can't stand eating alone in public, order room service instead.

Put a Ring on It

I didn't wait to get married to wear a wedding ring. I bought my own fake one about twenty years before I walked down the aisle. The reason single lady travelers should, in the immortal words of Beyoncé, put a ring on it is that the glittery band sends a subliminal message that you're unavailable. Jewelry won't stop a determined rapist, of course, but it might get you more respectful treatment from horny taxi drivers who think foreign women are sluts. It also might get you a better table at a restaurant. I still keep the decoy ring on while traveling, with the real one on the other hand because I can never keep track of which country wears wedding bands on which hand. (Some eastern European countries as well as Spain, Portugal, and Greece prefer the right hand.) If you're going to employ this ruse, ready a cover story about your bogus husband, in case anyone asks.

Hotel Safety

Several of my acquaintances have been sexually assaulted in their hotels. Other guests followed them into the elevator and then barged into their rooms. Hotel employees snuck in with keys. I think it's a good idea to get a door alarm. Hang this marvel on the doorknob, and satisfaction guaranteed. It lets off a godawful screech if an intruder tries to force his or her way into the room. The alarm costs around ten dollars online. Another variant, which can be slipped under the door, sounds off when the door opens. You'll sleep like a baby—until the alarm goes off.

For extra precaution, ask for a room on an upper floor and make sure the windows don't face out on a terrace, from which someone could climb in. (Ground-floor rooms are easier to break into from the outside.) But don't stay on a floor that's too high to jump from in case of fire. (Yes, a broken leg is unpleasant, but at least you'll survive.) If you smell smoke but can't flee the room safely, hang a sheet out the window to alert firefighters that someone is trapped in that room. Seek refuge in the bathroom. Fill the tub with water in order to wet towels and sheets and place them at the bottom of the doors to guard against smoke. Open windows and bathroom vents to air out the smoke.

As for break-ins, use every lock on the door. A Do Not Disturb sign that signals that the room is occupied might discourage a thief from barging in. Whatever you do, don't answer the door if you're not expecting anyone.

Hopefully, you will never face a terrorist assault like the one in Mumbai in 2008, when militants stormed two five-star hotels and held dozens of guests hostage. In such a situation, push furniture against the door and hide behind as many walls as possible.

As a general rule, don't ask for your room key in front of suspicious-looking people; if you must mention your room number, speak in a low voice that won't be heard by someone other than the receptionist. If you think you're being followed into an elevator, make an excuse about forgetting something and back out.

HEALTH EMERGENCIES THAT CAN RUIN A TRIP

Getting sick is never fun, especially when you're in a strange place where you may not speak the language. Before departing, identify reputable clinics in your destination. It's also worth arranging travel insurance for a medical evacuation, just in case. Most health insurance policies don't cover travel abroad, so you might need supplemental coverage. International SOS and Global Rescue are two of the world's largest medical travel services providers. Costs can run as low as three hundred dollars a year. Read the fine print, however, as some insurers won't cover emergencies that pertain to preexisting conditions or Ebola.

You might want to prearrange a Skype call with your doctor in case of crisis. Also, ask the hotel or U.S. consulate for a list of clinics or doctors. But be aware that the quality of care may not be equal to that to which you're accustomed (or maybe, if you get lucky, as I did in South Africa, it will surpass it). After suffering whiplash in a car in Russia, I saw a local doctor who prescribed keeping my neck immobile for weeks. The neck brace worsened the stiffness so badly that I required months of physical therapy in the United States to get my neck moving properly again. Before you go, ask an amenable doctor to prescribe all sorts of stuff for the medical kit that you can't get over the counter, like various broad-spectrum antibiotics for respiratory illness, wounds, the gut, and skin. Make sure the directions are clearly marked so that you don't take the digestive antibiotic for a skin infection, or vice versa. Failing stockpiling a collection of take-along pills, note your drug's generic and brand names and bring them to a local drugstore while you're traveling. A lot of foreign countries have friendly pharmacists who will dispense drugs that you'd otherwise need a prescription for in the United States. (Either they have prescribing powers or will do so regardless of the law—especially if, ahem, they can make a few bucks in the process.) However, double-check the English translation and recommended dosage, and inspect the packaging for dubious printing to make sure the drug is not counterfeit. Lots of companies and unscrupulous dealers dump drugs on Third World countries, so check that you're not taking medication that's gone bad, and by all means know what it contains. Politely refrain from buying if the package has been opened, in order to ensure that the pharmacist has not slipped in a different medicine in order to make a quick buck.

One time, my blood-compatible husband and I were en route to visit friends in Colombia with our three-year-old, who had never been on a long flight before. He panicked from claustrophobia and hollered so loudly that the pilot got on the intercom to ask for a child developmental expert on board. ("If so, please make yourself known to the flight attendants *immediately*.") No one appeared, alas, so we spent the rest of the flight fruitlessly trying to comfort the traumatized kid and profusely apologizing to everyone on board. Not wanting to repeat this distressing episode on the return flight, we went to the pharmacist in the small town where we were vacationing and asked (or, rather, begged) for a magic pill to help a toddler sleep. "I have just the thing," the helpful pharmacist said, handing over a little white box. "Give him one, and he'll sleep like a baby." Boy, did he. Like a dead baby. The kid was so still that we feared he'd stopped breathing.

After establishing a faint pulse, we worried that he might be brain damaged if or when he finally stirred to life. I don't know what was in that vial. The box wasn't clearly marked, and I didn't follow the advice I've just dispensed to you to take care when buying medication overseas. I took these desperate measures because I feared being seen as the worst mother in the Western Hemisphere. I didn't want to offend any more fellow passengers, and being cheap, I didn't want to pay for psychotherapy later on. It could be that the medicine was too potent for a small person. Or maybe it had expired. Our cherished son eventually woke up, and he developed into a healthy young adult without any signs of permanent impairment. But I wouldn't wish that experience, or that risk, on any parent—or anyone else, for that matter. Try to get the pills at home before you depart. And earplugs, too. You could go all Clooney and hand out noise-canceling headphones to fellow passengers on the plane, as George and

Amal did when they traveled with their twin babies. But that might require being, well, George and Amal Clooney.

Women's Health

Gather a group of women travelers together, and the talk will invariably turn to, um, our special needs while on the road. Yeast infections come up a lot, as do cystitis and other UTIs. New climates and water that upset the body's pH can promote candidiasis or urinary tract infections. Sitting long hours on airplanes or in wet bathing suits creates the perfect breeding ground. As with blisters, go on the offensive before the enemy strikes. Wear cotton underwear and loose trousers, and pack over-the-counter remedies. These would be Monistat for thrush and Uristat for urinary tract discomfort. Also, ask your doctor to proactively prescribe Diflucan for yeast. Upon returning, see a doctor if symptoms persist once the medication has run its course. You might have misdiagnosed yourself and need a prescription drug.

In case of sexual assault, find out before you travel whether and where you can obtain the morning-after pill and antiretrovirals. Also, contemplate how you'd handle the psychological repercussions of an attack. Who would you turn to for emotional support? A colleague who was raped in Russia went through contortions to find a doctor who could provide the medication in a timely fashion. It wasn't readily available, so she had to get on a plane to another country, several hours away. It was a horrific and upsetting experience, to say the least.

The Runs

Strange water in a strange country can upset even a strong stomach. The places I tend to travel to provide plenty of opportunities to get the runs due to unsanitary conditions, but a digestive tract can become upset anywhere. My travel bag always contains ample supplies of Imodium and chewable Pepto-Bismol, even if I'm only taking an Amtrak to Boston. Ask your doctor for a prescription for Zofran, an antinausea and vomiting medication that's helpful in case of food poisoning. For prevention, I slather on hand purifiers and drink bottled water. For really unsanitary places, where sewage gets mixed into what comes out of the tap, I'll pack water-purifying tablets or a filter wand, both of which can be ordered online.

Antibiotics

I always ask my doctor for a supply of antibiotics just in case I succumb to sinusitis or another infection. Searching for a local doctor abroad wastes valuable work and sightseeing time, as well as money. My internist recommends the general-purpose Zithromax Z-Pak or doxycycline. These medications are used to treat a wide variety of bacterial infections, including skin, ear, urinary, and respiratory infections. As a further precaution, I pack ciprofloxacin for gastrointestinal ailments, but be aware that bacteria have built up resistance to many types of antibiotics. Or, you may in fact have a viral infection, which wouldn't be cured by these meds.

Foot Notes

Whether on the job or on vacation, I'm on my feet all the time. And I've endured some horrendous foot blisters. And you usually realize you have them only when it's too late. The largest, most unpleasant and unsightly blister developed in Rwanda. I had to get there in a hurry to cover a breaking story, which didn't leave me time to break in my new pair of boots. Much as I love the Eccos, they require dedicated time to be broken in. The airport didn't sell the moleskin pads that I normally bring just in case, so you can guess what happened. The chafing Gore-Tex created blisters on my heels the diameter of golf balls. After just one day, walking in the boots became an agony. And the thick bandages I applied didn't help as barriers between the raw flesh and the shoes. I spent the rest of the assignment slipping about in flip-flops, which are not ideal footwear in refugee camps. I got hookworm walking across feces-strewn ground. You can get this parasite or a fungus from strolling in ordinary gardens or streets, so this isn't just a war-related problem. Since that fateful trip, I proactively apply antiblister balm or heel pads before going for a long walk in new shoes. I also pack antifungus cream that can treat skin ailments like ringworm and athlete's foot.

Toothaches

I'm not sure what's worse, having a painful toothache on vacation or seeing a foreign dentist with dirty hands. Generally, a toothache is the start of an infection, so reach for the antibiotics. As with the feet, prevention is the best approach. Before traveling, get a checkup and a cleaning. Floss and brush religiously while on the road, and rinse with bottled water. And use hand sanitizer before sticking your hands anywhere near your mouth. If you absolutely have to see a dentist, ask the U.S. consulate or hotel for recommendations.

Prescription Medication

If you have a life-threatening condition like diabetes that requires medication, think carefully about what would happen if you lost or ran out of your medication while traveling. Can you easily replace it, or get your doctor to phone a prescription into a foreign pharmacy? Probably not, in most cases. If you plan to be away for a long spell, call your health insurance company about getting a vacation override, so you can stock up on pills. Bring a big stash, to be stored in the carry-on luggage, in case your checked baggage is lost or delayed.

If you take commonly prescribed medications, consult the State Department's website to ascertain whether the drug is permitted in the destination country. (See Resources.) Possession of EpiPens, contraceptives, controlled substances such as opioids, and attention deficit medication such as Adderall or Ritalin could lead to the pills' confiscation and even your imprisonment in some places. Japan is particularly strict about stimulants, even over-the-counter medications. The State Department recommends having your doctors write a letter, translated into the host language and certified, with their contact information and credentials, your diagnosis, the treatment dosage details, and your full name and passport number.

Mosquitoes

More people die from mosquitoes than from war. The list of mosquito-borne diseases includes malaria, dengue fever, Zika, West Nile fever, yellow fever, Chikungunya, and encephalitis, to name a few. Even if you don't expire, you'll suffer one of the worst bouts of headache, fever, joint pain, and nausea in your life (which will feel like it is ebbing away). What with increasingly wetter climates in parts of the United States and elsewhere, scientists predict we'll see a profusion of mosquito-carried ailments in the years to come, especially dengue. In 2019 alone, three American states saw an outbreak of a rare form of encephalitis that killed five people. As it is, each year about 1,700 Americans return from travel overseas infected by the malarial parasite spread by these insects. I've had mild versions of malaria twice, and the shakes and nausea are no fun. On top of the debilitating headache come chills, diarrhea, vomiting, fever, sweating, and body aches. Worse, the parasite can stay in the system for weeks, if not years. Twenty years on, I still get occasional flare-ups when run down. The cerebral variety of malaria can prove fatal.

Wearing the proper clothes (not slapping) is the best way to get mosquitoes away from your body—long sleeves, thick socks, long pants, a hat. In the Siberian summer, which I discovered is surprisingly prone to clouds of bugs due to the thawing tundra, people wear hats with nets to guard their faces. They resemble beekeeper headgear. To ward off these pests during my travels, I bought repellant-saturated shirts and trousers at a camping store. These beauties retain the repellant even after several washings. They look terrible, but who cares what a malarial mosquito thinks?

However, just wearing protective clothes won't provide full protection. Nor will the added barriers of mosquito nets and coils and insect repellants applied to clothing as well as skin and even hair. The Centers for Disease Control and Prevention (CDC) recommends medicinal prophylactics, taken before, during, and after visits to a malarial zone in, say, vacation spots in South Africa, Mexico, and, believe it or not, parts of Italy. Here it gets tricky, because there are as many varieties of antimalarial meds to choose from as there are brands of toothpaste: Atovaquone/proguanil (brand name: Malarone), chloroquine (Aralen), mefloquine (Lariam), hydroxychloroquine (Plaquenil), primaquine, and doxycycline. Still, none of these will offer 100 percent fortification, especially against clever parasites that have developed resistance to particular strains in some regions. Most places have chloroquine-resistant parasites these days. The CDC publishes lists of which preventive to take in which area. Given the ever-changing nature of drug resistance, make sure you look at the latest version of the list.

In case these precautions fail, or you failed to follow them, some doctors will prescribe a potent medicine, sulfadoxine/pyrimethamine, sold under the brand name Fansidar, for you to take when symptoms appear. This advice comes with a caveat. According to Drugs.com, "Fansidar should be given with caution to patients with impaired renal or hepatic function, to those with possible folate deficiency and to those with severe allergy or bronchial asthma. As with some sulfonamide drugs, in glucose-6-phosphate dehydrogenase-deficient individuals, hemolysis may occur."

I'm not sure what that means, but I've heard reports of horrible vertigo, bizarre nightmares, rashes, and, in extreme cases, temporary insanity due to Fansidar. Urban legend in Africa holds that a guy experiencing a Fansidar reaction walked into the moving blades of a helicopter propeller. I couldn't confirm the story, but decided not to push my luck after experiencing weird Fansidar dreams. Flying giraffes with giant incisors ran after me across the savannah, and then a poisonous tarantula with a French accent picked up the chase. The next night, I dreamt that terrorists wearing Halloween masks and drooling blood broke into my hotel room. Normally I wake up before dying in nightmares, but in both these dreams, the attackers succeeded in killing me. While this may strike you as routine, you have to understand that when traveling on assignment, I normally have dull dreams about doing my laundry. The most dangerous thing that ever occurred in these dreams was my accidentally putting bleach into the dark wash. So, the Fansidar assassins freaked me out. I threw the pills away in the morning, wagering that it was better to power through malarial fever than to die each night.

Please consider the following when weighing antimalarial options: You can swallow only so many preventive pills before they damage the body. I've taken so many prophylactics over the decades that my doctor now warns that any more will "insult" my liver. I will not allow a mosquito pill to insult my liver. No one is allowed to insult my organs but me and Mr. Merlot. That means going back to square one: Cover the body, burn coils, put up nets, or just stay home.

Many people have asked what to do if they haven't had routine vaccinations for highly contagious diseases that have basically been eliminated in the United States, such as measles and mumps. Well, it's simple: If you're going somewhere where infectious illnesses are endemic, get the darned shots. Otherwise, don't travel. If you contract the sickness abroad, you then can infect other people who similarly resisted vaccination. The most recent measles outbreaks in the United States were caused by someone traveling overseas who then brought it back. Don't be one of these jerks who endanger others, particularly children.

CASH IS KING

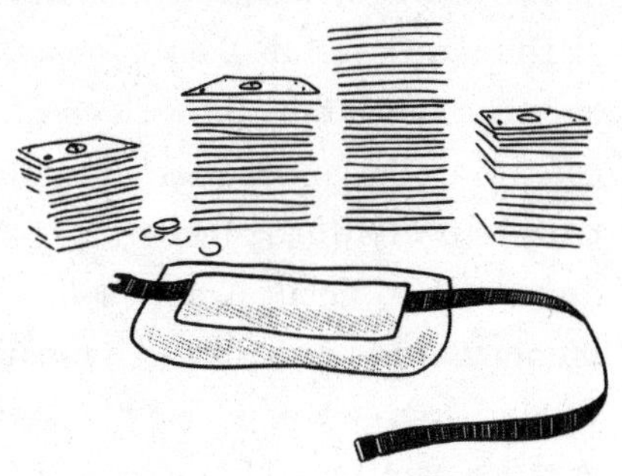

Finances require the same sort of foresight as choosing a hotel. I normally change money upon arriving at the airport, and thereafter withdraw cash from ATMs or exchange it at banks or accredited exchange centers, always looking over my shoulder to make sure some goon isn't going to stick me up. In order to reduce the chance of muggings, visit the ATM during the day, on a well-trafficked street. Also keep your bank's emergency number on hand to call in case your card is lost or stolen. An ATM machine in Norway ate my card, which taught me to get out money during business hours. It being nighttime, the bank was closed, and I had to wait until the next day for the manager to call a tech to retrieve the card. Much to the consternation of the photographer I was traveling with, I had a Plan B: borrow *his* card.

If you're getting money out of a local ATM or using a credit card, beware of fraud. My husband went to Caracas for a conference and used his credit card for hotel expenses. He didn't leave the hotel because he was under surveillance by the Venezuelan government the entire time. A month later, mysterious charges from a Coconut Club on El Yaque beach mysteriously appeared on our Visa bill. The club receives high ratings on TripAdvisor.com by "Bertvone" of Geneva for its "most confortable [*sic*] beach bed." It doesn't get high ratings in my household. Someone who stole my husband's identity was living *la vida loca* there, ordering twelve thousand dollars' worth of drinks at the old Coconut. Lucky for us, the friendly folks in Visa's fraud department noticed something was up and canceled the charge. However, for added protection, they also froze our credit card whenever we subsequently traveled anywhere in Latin America. I routinely go to Mexico on business and was stuck in a most unfortunate position in Ciudad Juárez when Visa blocked me from paying my bill at the Fiesta Inn. That's the sort of thing the U.S. consulate doesn't help you with. Henceforth, we always alerted the credit card companies to upcoming foreign travel well in advance. I suggest you do, too. And out of loyalty to me, don't patronize the Coconut Club.

Because I often travel to countries where the banking system has collapsed, or never really took off, cash reigns. Across Africa, I routinely carried twenty thousand dollars to cover three months' worth of expenses and emergency funds. Being a human Citibank branch meant I had to find a way to stash this fortune safely. Enter, with fanfare, the money belt! But not just any money belt. I endorse an ingenious money belt that acts like a belt, sliding through the pant loops, as opposed to those impractical things that strap around the neck or fit under clothes. The first is ridiculous—anyone could cut the cords and run off with it. The second entails rummaging around in your pants each time you want to pay for a Coke. Worse, it sticks out like a colostomy bag. The belt I'm talking about is made of leather or nylon webbing. It's truly amazing how many bills you can squeeze into these things if the money is folded tightly enough. Some folks use pocket socks for bigger items like passports and credit cards. I know women who have hidden cash inside sanitary napkins. They make a slit in the cotton and slip the money in. That has too much of a yuck factor for me, but I'm not passing judgment on anyone who wants to try it.

While you're folding the bills (wherever you decide to store them), check that they are crisp and of a certain vintage. Lots of places in the world won't accept crinkled or ripped moneys; Nigeria, for instance, for a while rejected dollar bills printed before 2006. I've had shopkeepers in Portugal reject bills because they were torn at the corner or scribbled on. As with everything else in this book, research the matter before traveling.

Once you've got the money, walk around with only the cash and credit/debit cards you actually need. Also, spread your cash around. Have a few bills in your pocket in case you're held up or need to bribe someone quickly, and leave whatever you don't need in the hotel safe or somewhere exceedingly secure where no one would think of looking. Some women swear by hiding money at the bottom of a tampon box or in their dirty laundry, but that might not discourage a determined thief.

One Last Thing

For sure, people pick up traveler's bugs from bad food, but you know what really spreads gastro parasites? Money, handled by people who don't wash their hands properly. Generously apply hand sanitizer after any financial transaction.

RULES OF THE ROAD: CONSIDERATIONS FOR PLANES, TRAINS, AND AUTOMOBILES

Ever show up in a strange city and not know your way around? Everybody does that. That's the definition of "strange city"! I do it all the time, frequently in locales that don't have tarmac roads or city maps. I don't like to use long-distance public transport like buses unless absolutely necessary. Granted, a bus or train provides the opportunity to meet the locals, and suffer like they do. But a bus or train or minivan robs you of the ability to control your movements when the vehicle is stormed by hostage takers or breaks down at the edge of a cliff. To save time, and worry, I rely on Uber (if it exists in that country) and taxis. Or I rent cars with drivers. Normally someone at the hotel front desk will know a guy with a car, most likely his cousin. Hiring a driver means you don't have to contend with bewildering local traffic rules. Case in point: A cop in Luanda pulled me over for failing to stop at a stoplight. When I pointed out that none existed, he stretched out his hand for a "fine" (read: bribe). "There used to be one," he said. "Pay up." Pro tip: Know the going rate for bribes so that you don't overpay. That's not something the State Department will tell you, but other travelers will.

Another pro tip: For a long-haul trip, no matter who is driving, kick the tires and rummage around in the machinery to make sure the vehicle is running properly. I'm speaking from experience. Over the years, I quickly learned that rented cars can break down or emit smoke for lack of tune-ups. Also, learn how to change tires, if you don't know already. If traveling in remote areas, the car should have certain essentials in case you get stuck overnight in the middle of nowhere, as I have on many occasions. These include the medical kit and ready-to-go bag from chapter 2 ("The Basics") as well as tow chains (stronger than ropes), wooden planks (for mud), a sleeping bag, tarp, rain gear, flares, a flashlight, a shovel, a jack, nonperishable food such as energy bars, spare water and petrol, and spare tires. (Yes, *tires* plural. On a family holiday in Swaziland, we busted three tires in one day. The roads resembled moon craters, and my husband drives blisteringly fast.)

Finally, a lot of countries don't accept American driver's licenses, or traffic cops there can't read what the document says. The American Automobile Association (AAA) helps get around this snafu by issuing an international driver's permit, to be used alongside the American license. A one-year permit costs only twenty-four dollars and serves as an accepted form of identification in 150 countries. It can be obtained at AAA offices or through the mail. Remember to pack your American license, too, as the permit doesn't serve as a substitute.

UBER SAFETY

IMPORTANT: Before getting into any hired car, check the license plate and make sure it matches the number and make of the car you're expecting. As a further precaution, use the "Share My Trip" function in the Uber app with a family member or friend. As the name suggests, it will share with a third party of your choice the driver's name, photo, license plate number, and location, and send them a text or notification that tracks your trip and ETA.

Also, sit in the backseat on the side away from traffic, which will enable an easier getaway should the driver turn out to be a creep.

Last, whatever car you ride in, don't forget to wear a seat belt!

OFF THE BEATEN PATH

Going off trail without a rescue plan is insane. Even a simple hike up a "safe" mountain to watch the sunset can lead to kids and adults wandering around in the wilderness unsure how to get home. Too many people go backpacking, skiing, etc., without proper preparation or exit strategies, unable to rely on GPS because their phones can't get reception and no one knows where they are. One can fall and get hurt anywhere, such as a parking lot at a strip mall. But the consequences of such a tumble can be fatal in a remote setting. Overriding safety concerns in my line of work involve reporters going off to break a story on their own with no regard for their safety. They fly to an exciting place like Somalia without the support of a major news organization, or without proper gear and a communication plan. This free-for-all approach hurts not only the adventurer in question but also those left behind: parents, significant others, not to mention the poor chump at the U.S. consulate who gets a call at 2 a.m. to inform him that an American has gone missing. I'm not saying one shouldn't stray off the path, but great care should be taken to ensure that the maximum safeguards are in place.

I see a correlation between irresponsible correspondents

and backpackers who intentionally stray into dodgy areas like war zones and disputed borders. Don't get me wrong. I love hiking. It's one of my favorite pastimes, as long as it's on flat-ish ground that doesn't cause altitude sickness. But I don't ramble around in shady places. By shady, I don't mean sunless. I mean where hostile groups lurk and Americans are assumed to be spies, or where I have to bushwhack a trail because no one has walked there in centuries. Consider the example of Patrick Braxton-Andrew, a high school Spanish teacher from North Carolina who took a stroll through Mexico's Copper Canyon on October 28, 2018, and went missing. Violent drug cartels operated in the region. His corpse was discovered later; he had been murdered by a dealer. Nine years earlier, three Americans were taken into custody by Iranian border guards for crossing into that country while hiking around its border with Iraqi Kurdistan. The trio was imprisoned and mistreated until their release two years later. Take heed from these examples. Trekking around lawless areas is asking for trouble, especially when going solo. Consult the Sierra Club for alternatives. The world brims with stunning landscapes that don't attract *bandidos*.

Even if you opt for the Appalachian Trail as opposed to the Iraqi border, accidents (e.g., broken legs and lightning strikes) can occur. To face such unpleasant eventualities with the utmost confidence, take a wilderness first aid course beforehand and carry a mini inReach satellite device. REI, the Red Cross, and a variety of private companies offer these courses, which can last anywhere from one day to a week. A satellite communicator is a combined GPS tracker, two-way messenger, navigation tool, and SOS device. (See Resources.)

TRAVEL COMPANIONS

Apropos, I always counsel journalists to travel with a buddy. That way, someone can call for help if you pass out or something more terrible happens. The companion can watch your back while you are taking photographs and negotiate with authorities when you're being arrested. Two's company, as they say—well, they should say "the *right* company." A bad-tempered travel mate can spoil a trip, whether it's for pleasure or business. Compatibility in humor, alcohol tolerance, and "adventure," otherwise known as great peril, determine a smooth ride. One particularly taxing photographer, who shall go unnamed, drove me so bats that I was ready to hand him over to kidnappers. He kept arguing with taxi drivers and refused to hand over his bags for inspection. He drank too much in the evenings, exhausted our budget by ordering the most expensive meat on the menu, and then pissed in the bath bucket. After that, I vetted my travel partners carefully and went only with people whose quirks I could tolerate. Also, I have a frank discussion with my traveling companion before we leave, about expectations and thresholds for risk. The same talk is needed for that friend of a friend who tags along on your backpacking trip in Europe. Aside from improving the enjoyment factor, this important discussion should establish whether it's cool to speak English loudly in the street or invite back to the Airbnb some guy you met at a nightclub.

TRAVEL WITH CHILDREN

It probably goes without saying that like cantankerous photojournalists, kids make for challenging travel companions. Much as we love them, the two groups have much in common. They want to do unwise things, like order ice from a street cart buzzing with flies or ride a moped without a helmet. Their complaints can wear you down and prompt you to make bad decisions just to appease them. Journalists have the attention span of three-year-olds, and similarly require constant hydration. Journalists balk at orders. The one difference is that we don't take up precious suitcase room with diapers, baby formula, dolls, puzzles, and sticker books.

The key for both demographics, I have found, is to make them believe they're getting the upper hand. Both kids and journalists love to break rules and then boast about it, so give them ample opportunity to think they are badasses without letting them actually do something stupid that could hurt someone. I'm no terrific mother (or a fun person to travel with, for that matter), but I will share one tip that worked with my then twelve-year-old son when I dragged him on an assignment to Mexico. I don't know if this will work for your children, but here goes.

The kid was understandably bored hanging out with his mother while she worked, so I had to dream up something to make the trip worthwhile, or at least tolerable. So I did what I would do with a colleague: I challenged him to a "Who Can Eat the Grossest Food?" contest. The disgusting things I have dared my friends to eat include sheep's eyeballs, cane rat, and my cooking. The prize for winning the competition with my kid wasn't extravagant, because I'm cheap, but the gross factor was enough of a motivator. We worked our way through grasshoppers, ants, worms, brain, armadillo, mosquito eggs, and tripe. He accidentally ate a fly that landed on his beef taco, and counted it for good measure. We were neck and neck until we hit an open-air market in Oaxaca, where a vendor waved a monstrous bug. It had bulging eyes and spindly legs, like the star of a horror movie. I wasn't going to put that repulsive thing in my mouth, but the kid rose to the occasion and *swallowed it*—with his eyes wide open. What pluck! The vendor lady offered him another, but he respectfully declined. Flush with fresh pride, my offspring took home souvenirs of ground crickets for his friend Henry, as well as tales of bravado—much like journalists and their war stories.

Aside from sampling revolting dishes, one should consider other practical steps to make the trip easier for all. To wit: Pack essential items like baby formula, wipes, snacks, and amusing toys in your hand luggage. And plan ahead for emergencies: tantrums. Explain the process of going through security before you get there, in order to prevent meltdowns on the TSA line. We neglected to do just this with our toddler while going through security for a flight to Bogotá, and he threw a fit when a strapping guard with a Galil automatic weapon grabbed his toy cat in order to put it through the X-ray machine. My son's epic outburst and the dirty looks from others on line still give me nightmares.

Once you've wrestled the child and stuffed animal onto the plane, pay special heed to emergency instructions so you'll know how to strap the oxygen mask onto Junior should the aircraft catch fire. Arrange to sit near an emergency exit to facilitate running off before the other passengers. Don't seat the wee ones on the aisle, as their little feet might get run over by the food cart. If the offspring is traveling unaccompanied, make abundantly clear to the airline that you *must* be advised if they are diverted to another airport. If the children don't have cell phones, make sure they can recite your telephone number by heart and that they know to insist to airline staff that they call you. Once, when my then ten-year-old son flew back alone from Mexico, the plane was diverted to Virginia for a few hours during a storm—and the airline didn't text or call us! While Anton was having the time of his life eating candy and playing games with the other equally stranded minors, we parents were freaking out.

As for documentation, American passports for kids expire quicker than adults' and have to be renewed more often. If your surname differs from the child's, carry proof that you're the guardian, such as a notarized letter from the other parent and a copy of the birth certificate, in order to ward off any suspicions of human trafficking. The TSA generally doesn't ask questions, but immigration on the other side might. An assertive officer at Ben Gurion Airport, in Israel, once demanded to know why my son was not a "Matloff." He noted that the kid did not have my Jewish nose. Once we had established that I was legit, he then noted the kid's age and asked if he was preparing for his bar mitzvah. I didn't think that was the man's business, but here's another tip for the savvy traveler: Always act polite at the immigration booth.

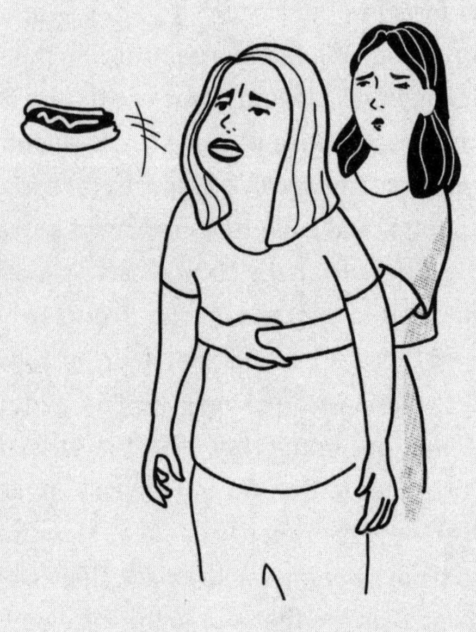

Chapter 4

JUST PLUG IT—EMERGENCY FIRST AID

A few years back, my friend Tina was at the top of the subway stairs at Thirty-Fourth Street in Manhattan when she noticed a crowd standing around a very large woman. The woman was choking to death. She had all the signs: purplish-red face, watery eyes. She couldn't speak and looked on the verge of collapse. Everyone just stood there watching, as if they knew they should do something but didn't know what. So, Tina, a badass war correspondent who thrives in crisis situations, figured she should try the Heimlich, which she'd learned many years earlier, in the Girl Scouts. She walked behind the woman, wrapped her arms around the woman's belly, and pushed upward, as she'd been taught. Nothing. Then she did it again, this time super hard, and voilà! A very large chunk of hot dog flew across the sidewalk and landed in the street. The victim stopped choking. Tina asked someone in the crowd to hand over his soft drink for the woman, who was exhausted but kept saying "thank you" over and over, and she told the lady to chew her food better in the future. The crowd clapped, and our intrepid correspondent went on her way.

Let's be clear. First aid isn't about your being a hero. It's about your being a *first responder.* The reason I'm telling you this story is that war correspondents routinely learn how to plug bullet holes and set fractures in case someone around them gets hurt. Unless we're embedded with a military unit with medics, we're often far from clinics, which are rudimentary at best, so we carry medical kits with items such as tourniquets and ointments. Little-known fact: Journalists are more likely to die from car accidents than ballistics, so we have to be prepared to handle mundane eventualities like shock or heart attacks.

As my pal Tina so ably demonstrated, first aid skills come in handy not just for conflict situations but also on vacation or when you're walking down the street minding your own business. Everyone, from eighth-graders to adults, would benefit from such training. In these times of mass shootings, we should all know how to stanch bleeding until the medics reach the scene. Bystanders are the best first responders because they are right on the spot before the ambulance can arrive. For example, it was bystanders who intervened to stabilize the wounded before ambulances arrived at both the Boston Marathon bombing site in 2013 and the 2017 Las Vegas shooting. In Boston, thanks to passersby's improvised tourniquets and the application of pressure, no victim who got to a hospital afterward died. Another fact: About a quarter of emergency department visits could be avoided with the application of basic first aid on the scene. Many people survive no matter what, but intervening quickly could help preserve their quality of life. Rapid first aid might save them from having to use diapers for the rest of their lives or from never remembering their kids' names.

Just knowing how to tend to the injured will steady everyone, including yourself and the guy who just got shot in the leg or broke it falling down a hill. When pandemonium breaks out, you can add to that chaos or help calm it down. Obviously, you'll want to calm it down. Most people say, "I'm afraid to do the wrong thing." That's probably what the people standing around the spluttering woman at the top of those subway steps were thinking. Yet, if you're sure of your skills and have gotten some training through, say, the Red Cross, the National Safety Council, or Stop the Bleed, you'll take action and do the right thing. (See Resources.) The intensive wilderness first aid courses mentioned in the last chapter provide training for a wider swath of emergencies than run-of-the-mill CPR training. Responding correctly will become instinctive, like holding your breath underwater. If you have the confidence that you know what to do, then you'll be 50 percent more likely to make the situation better. It's important to take refreshers once you receive the training. (We advise journalists to do so yearly.) Skills grow fuzzy over time, and medicine is dynamic. What doctors recommended twenty years ago, like keeping a concussed person awake, may not be considered the best practice today.

The following are some insights into what to do in various emergency situations. It's impossible to list every possible scenario, which is what makes being prepared so challenging and even scary. This catalog is by no means exhaustive; instead, it's representative of the type of circumstances that are common but that might not occur to a lot of people. I'm not covering stuff like CPR and airway obstruction, which you can learn in an everyday Red Cross course. I'm also leaving the question of ice-versus-heat for minor injuries to your kid's sports coach. But first, a disclaimer: Do not—I repeat, do *not*—head into a crisis scene and start attending to bodies based on having read this chapter. Know what you're doing and call 911 regardless. My intention here is to orient you toward what to look for in case of emergency and how to approach it. Do not try any of these procedures at home, or at a concert, or at church, or at a traffic light, without taking a proper first aid course. A lot of the moves involve muscle memory, and you need to practice them over and over, not just rely on pictures or words. The list is far from exhaustive, but covers some of the essential principles our medical trainers teach correspondents, which are vital for civilian life, too.

SCOPE THE SCENE

Before anything else, assess the situation. Some people's instinctual response when they witness a shooting or see a dead body is "I'm going in." That's fine in principle, but not always wise. Pausing can feel excruciating, but if you don't pay attention—if the active shooter is lingering nearby, or if the terrorist with the butcher knife is lurking behind a tree—you might die. Take a minute to look around the scene. Keep your head on swivel and survey the landscape. Has the gunfire stopped? Is the driver who just plowed through protesters still in his car? If so, hold back. Consider your personal safety first. Your first instinct should never—I repeat, *never*—be to run toward danger. It should be to run and hide. You have to make sure you're safe before helping others. We war correspondents have a saying: A dead journalist is a useless journalist. Same with civilians.

FIELD TRIAGE

Triage is the process of sorting victims in a battle or disaster to determine their medical priority in order to increase the number of survivors. The term came into use among eighteenth-century coffee growers, who sorted beans into best, middling, and broken. One day, you may find yourself not sorting beans, but evaluating which victim needs the most urgent care following a car crash, a climbing accident in the wilderness, or a sports event stampede.

Let's say, for example, that you're at a concert and a deranged man opens fire on the crowd. The shooter eventually shoots himself, at which point it's okay to crawl to the four wounded people around you. One has been shot in the head and is unresponsive. The second has blood streaming from his shoulder, but is able to answer questions through gritted teeth. A third person is trying to stanch bleeding in his groin area and is growing weak. The fourth has a broken tibia (shinbone) sticking out of her flesh.

You can't attend to all of them simultaneously. So, whom do you treat first?

Answer: The groin injury victim. Bleeding, shock, and airway obstruction are the three main killers, so anyone who has severe signs of one of these will die without emergency assistance. The shoulder is an extremity, so that wound is less serious. You may not be able to save the unresponsive man with the bullet to the head, especially if his breathing is slowing down. Monitor him closely; ditto for the woman with the tibia break if she starts to lose a lot of blood. But the person with the most life-threatening crisis with the highest survival probability goes first.

CALL A VET!

Sometimes there's no doctor or hospital close by. If that's the case, and someone needs urgent medical attention, ask for the nearest veterinarian. Seriously. Vets know how to set fractures and clean up and sew wounds. Dogs or donkeys aren't that different from humans when you get down to it. They have bones and flesh, and they bleed, too. In a pinch, a good vet can save a life.

SHOCK

Shock occurs when there is not enough pressure for blood and oxygen to reach the brain and organs. Blood loss and dehydration cause shock. You'll die if you lose a liter of fluids over one hour without replenishing it. Indeed, shock from diarrhea is one of the biggest killers in the developing world. Shock takes many forms, and can result as well from sugar lows (if the person is diabetic), sepsis, severe dehydration, and allergies. The most common symptom is dramatically low blood pressure, so if a pale person looks like they're about to pass out or already have, rush them to the emergency room. If the person is diabetic and has missed a meal, you might be able to stabilize them with glucose tablets or a high-sugar snack like candy or orange juice, but proceed to the hospital if symptoms worsen. Just to make your life and the patient's difficult, the symptoms of shock can vary widely depending on what's causing it. The gamut of signs includes: rapid heart rate, trouble breathing, slow pulse, fever, sweating, clammy skin, confusion, nausea, vomiting, swelling, shaking, dizziness, and fainting.

DRESS FOR SUCCESS

Don't forget latex gloves, in case the patient has HIV or another disease that can be passed through bodily fluids. I generally walk around with gloves in my bag. You never know when you're going to stumble upon an accident scene, and the gloves weigh less than a pack of gum. They're also great when you're walking the dog and have forgotten plastic bags to pick up the poop.

BRAIN INJURY

Don't mess with the brain. It will mess with you back. If a person complains of a wicked headache, can't retain new information, and/or loses consciousness, they probably have a brain injury. If they ask the same thing over and over, that's a brain injury. Don't be too worried about a gash to the head, unless the skull and brain are exposed. Brain failure occurs when the brain swells and can't get enough oxygen. Signs include a projectile vomit-o-rama and extreme sensitivity to light and sound. Another sign is an icepick-is-jabbing-me headache worse than any migraine, the type of pain that jumps off the one-to-ten scale. If symptoms come on within minutes, get moving toward a hospital. (If, however, the headache develops over four hours, you have time.) Contrary to past common wisdom, let the patient sleep or rest for a day, like a mushroom in a cool, dark zone. If they have seizures, don't hold them down, as that could break bones, including yours. Place a pillow under their head, and contrary to what you've seen on TV, don't stick things like a finger in their mouth, as it might get chewed off. Afterward, clean out the foam, any broken teeth, and bits of bitten tongue to make sure they don't choke on them.

OVERDOSES

Narcotics are generally not the poison of journalists. Being tethered to barstools, we're more likely to suffer from liver damage or embarrassing drunken antics. I recall one particularly wild party in Mexico where an inebriated reporter fell out a window. (He emerged unscathed and provided endless dinner party stories for the rest of us.) But given the severity of the opioid crisis in America, a growing number of people taking my safety workshops ask about treatment for overdoses. The majority of ODs are from fentanyl, which is increasingly being added to cocaine, Ecstasy, and other recreational drugs without buyers' knowledge.

Call 911 if you see an unresponsive person with pale, clammy skin; a slow heartbeat; labored breathing; and blue lips and nails. Just to be sure they're not sleeping or drunk, brusquely rub your knuckles into the chest muscles. The patient will stir to life if it's not an overdose. While waiting for emergency responders, administer naloxone, also sold as Narcan, which you can get over the counter at pharmacies in forty-six states. I can obtain the spray without a prescription at my local Rite Aid, and I often carry around a supply just in case. It's a cinch to use—either follow the directions or take a free course (see Resources)—and is effective when administered quickly.

Clear the person's mouth first, to make sure there's nothing choke-worthy like vomit in there. (This is another instance in which latex gloves come in handy. It's unpleasant and of dubious safety to stick your hand into a barf-filled mouth.) If the person is puking, roll them to their left side so the vomit doesn't get stuck in the airway. The medication is sprayed up the nose. Tilt the head back and squirt it into one nostril. Repeat in two to five minutes if the person overdosing doesn't take a deep breath or sit up groggily. If they've stopped breathing, hope that the ambulance gets there soon. Otherwise, administer CPR and more naloxone.

BLOOD AND GORE

Severed Parts

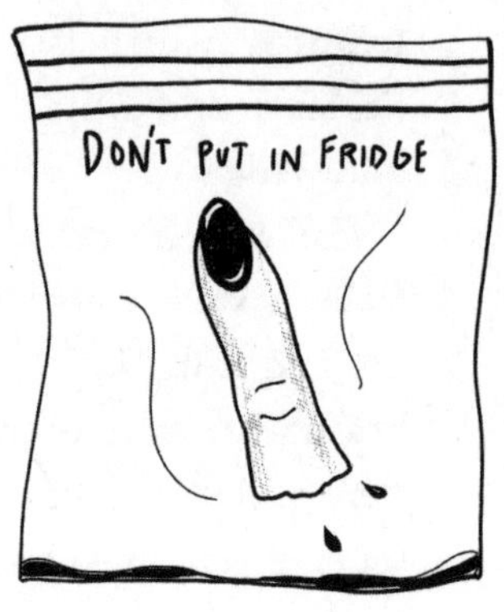

As our medical trainer, Sawyer Alberi, points out, people like to keep their severed parts with them. Makes them feel safer knowing their limb or digit is right nearby. If your or someone else's fingers have just gotten cut off, store them in a Ziploc bag. Keep them moist and cool but not drenched. This goes for spilled intestines as well. I heard a sad story about an acquaintance who lost a finger parachuting. It stayed behind when he jumped out of the plane. When he landed, the first thing he asked for was that finger; he wanted it reattached. Unfortunately, someone had put it on ice, thinking that would preserve it. But a finger is not an oyster. Ice damages tissue. So, make sure there's no ice in the Ziploc bag.

Rare Blood Types

I like to travel with my personal blood bank. For me, that means my husband, who shares my blood type. Knowing that my beloved could cough up a few liters of his own supply provided endless peace of mind when I hemorrhaged from a miscarriage in Russia, losing about a liter of blood. The incident also convinced me that blood compatibility should be established for all couples either contemplating marriage or just swiping right on dating apps. It's more important than similar tastes in music or a sense of humor. People with the rare Rh-negative blood type have died after receiving transfusions of the wrong blood. This can be easily avoided by choosing the proper life partner and making sure they are next to you 24/7.

However, in case this is not possible (or desirable), or if you insist on dating someone who is Rh positive when you're Rh negative, then you need to make serious provisions when traveling to a country where your blood type is rare. The universal donor type is O negative, which means anyone can tolerate it, but in some hospitals, it's in short supply. You can find out your type by asking your doctor or a health center/blood donation center to do a test. Or you can order one online (see Resources). The test costs about ten dollars and takes just a few minutes to complete. Some people wear bracelets or necklaces with their info. My father, who had an extremely rare blood type, wore one in World War II. Fortunately, he never got wounded, but it made him feel more secure (or as secure as one could feel when under Nazi mortar fire). You could get an attractive chain in silver or gold, to match other jewelry. Others prefer to keep on their person an emergency card, written in the local language, with their blood information and that of local clinics that have a supply. Check the organization Rhesus Negative. Its Web page (see Resources) links the user to other Rh-negative-related groups around the world. Hopefully, if you're brought unconscious to a hospital, someone will think to look at the card and get you the right blood.

External Bleeding

Bleeding occurs from all sorts of injuries: stab wounds, gunshots, car crashes, animal bites. The car door severs a finger.

A nail is driven into the hand. A stray dog tears at one's thigh. A wine bottle smashes to the floor. Ouch, my bare foot! The thing about external bleeding is that, for better or worse, it eventually stops. In severe circumstances, though, it takes less than a minute to lose the equivalent of two water bottles full of blood. This brings one perilously close to the jaws of death. You need to turn off the faucet, as it were, by applying pressure until the blood can clot and prevent even more from leaking out. Direct pressure stops 90 percent of external bleeds. Tourniquets control bleeding in extremities by cutting off all circulation. If you don't have one handy, one can be improvised with something bulky, like a scarf or T-shirt, tied right above the wound. Put a stick or pencil in the knot and twist it to apply more pressure. Don't use a thin belt, which can cut into flesh. A really thick one might do. (Fashion choices count!) You know it's tight enough when the blood stops dripping. I often hear the question "How do you know it's too tight?" Let's be clear, tourniquets are not comfortable, but you'll know circulation has been cut off when the patient complains of pins and needles and the fingers or toes turn white and cold. Provided that the tourniquet is not too tight, it's safe to leave it on for a couple of hours or until the patient can get to a doctor (or vet).

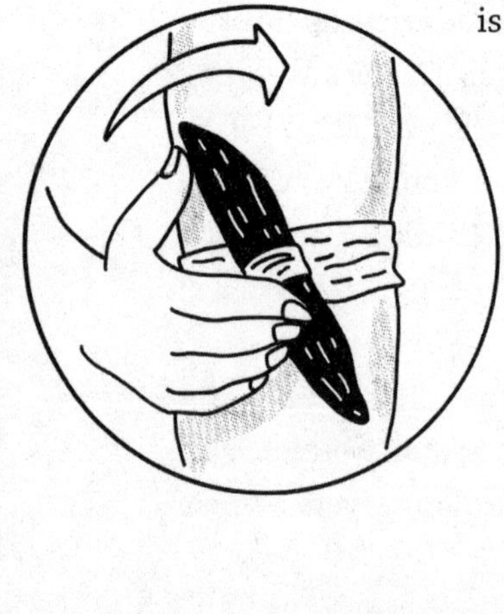

The victim will likely be freaking out, despite your excellent tourniquet-tying technique, so give them a job to do. Tell them to put pressure on the wound, which will not only help stabilize the situation but also distract them from the gore.

Whatever happens, remain composed. If you exude calm, they'll be more likely to relax and accept that they are not going to die just yet. Don't remove the tourniquet or loosen it, even if the patient continues to complain. Use a second one if blood is still leaking out. It might cause some nerve damage, but there is no point at which a tourniquet will cause death. Also, mark the time the tourniquet was put on, so that when the patient gets to the hospital, the staff will know how long circulation has been cut off.

Bleeding from vessels under the armpit or in the groin area is more complicated to treat than bleeding in the extremities. You can't tie a tourniquet around the femoral artery, which is lodged deep in the groin area. So, you need to reach inside the wound, feel around for spurting blood and warmth, and put pressure on that spot. Once the squirting movement slows down, stuff the wound with gauze. Again, be matter-of-fact when you stick your hand inside someone. Do not be deterred if the victim screams, "She just put her hand inside my pelvis!" I've never had the pleasure of putting this into practice, but my formidable medical instructor, Alberi, has; she's done medic tours in Afghanistan and offers this sage advice: "Just say, 'Saving your life,' and carry on. Once you pack the wound and wrap dressing around it, I promise he'll thank you."

In our workshops, Alberi pumps fake blood into dead chickens, and trainees stick their hands in the glutinous cavity to practice dressing wounds. She mixes red dye with hair gel to simulate the lifeblood inside someone's pelvis. It feels gross at first, like a slimy corpse with pulsating goo—which is exactly what it is—but after a few attempts, the sensation and detecting the motion become routine. Trainees say they come away with a decreased appetite for rotisseries but also a tremendous sense of mastery over stuffing Thanksgiving turkeys. Well, not everyone. Once we had a guy who refused to put his hand inside the chicken. He was worried about getting the fake blood on his new suede loafers. We told him to avoid war zones.

Internal Bleeding

Unlike wounds that gush blood outside the body, bleeding within the body can be harder for the layperson to diagnose. Signs of an internal bleed can include dizziness, unbearable pain in the stomach or other organ, passing out, shock, a plummeting blood pressure, and bloody vomit or diarrhea. If organs are hemorrhaging, do not exert pressure or try to resolve the problem yourself. This is one for the emergency room.

EXTREME AVERSION TO BLOOD

Along a similar, um, vein, don't go to scenes of car accidents or even to butcher shops if you faint at the sight of blood. Seriously. If you pass out while shopping for veal or after cutting yourself while chopping onions, you could inconvenience or even endanger those who have to revive you. A photographer who worked in trouble spots around the globe who took one of our courses in New York City fainted while watching the first aid slideshow of gruesome injuries. We heard a thump and then noticed her sprawled unconscious on the floor. Fortunately, the medics, being medics, knew just what to do and revived her in no time. They got her limp body to sit up and put her head on her knees. When she came to, they offered her a cup of water and asked her probing questions to ensure she wasn't concussed. Once the fainter had sufficiently regained her composure, we had a heart-to-heart talk about her changing careers (and going vegetarian).

HOW TO DRAG A BODY

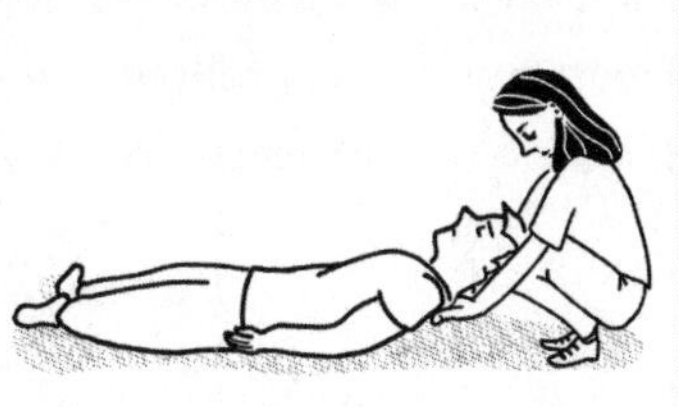

HOW TO DRAG A BODY

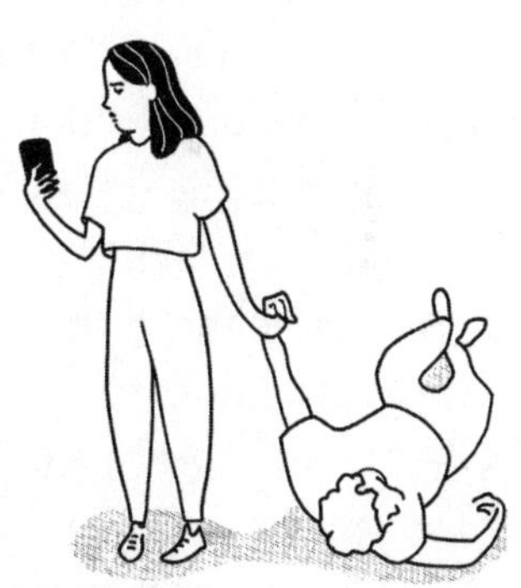

HOW NOT TO DRAG A BODY

The rule of thumb is to wait until first responders arrive, because moving an injured person the wrong way can paralyze them or worsen whatever damage they've suffered, be it to the spine, bones, or brain. However, if it looks like the emergency workers aren't arriving anytime soon and the victim appears to be facing fatal injury, it's better to take action.

So, what's the appropriate action? Shift them into as flat a position as possible, pulling the shirt above the shoulders on both sides of the head to prevent the head from rolling. If the victim is vomiting or choking on blood, roll them onto their side with the help of someone else, to prevent bending the neck and body. Whatever you do, make sure to stabilize them. Then wait until help arrives.

BROKEN BONES

Suspected fractures should be splinted and/or immobilized. Splints can be fashioned from a surprising number of items, including cardboard and sticks. Use cloth, clothing, or climbing rope to secure the splint, taking care all the while not to cut off circulation by too tight a wrap. Be especially gentle if a bone is sticking out. Look for signs of major bleeding; if you find them, follow the instructions under "External Bleeding" or "Internal Bleeding."

INFECTION

An infection can set in as early as twenty-four hours after someone is shot or cut, but it usually takes about seven to ten days. Signs of infection are murky fluid, soreness, and swelling around the wound site. Neosporin or an over-the-counter triple antibiotic is good for minor infections. So is cleaning the wound with potable water and applying garlic and turmeric. But these won't help with bad stuff like foul pus, fever, vomiting, abdominal pain, and severe malaise that worsen by the day. Serious infections may lead to sepsis and require oral antibiotics and a trip to the doctor—fast. If there's none nearby, then—you guessed it—call a vet.

BURNS

Let's myth-bust here. People smear all sorts of things on burns: butter, oil, mayonnaise, salt. No, no, no, and no! Keep all these cooking ingredients away from scorched skin. Salt should be a no-brainer. (Ouch!) And there's no evidence that the other kitchen substances will help healing; in fact, they might contain harmful bacteria that could lead to infection. Maybe apply a dab of aloe vera to keep the burn moist. It soothes and shouldn't cause any harm. Whatever you do, ice does not belong on a burn. It can cause further injury and even frostbite. Cool, not cold, running water is okay for very minor burns, but never for anything serious.

RABIES, VENOM, AND ANIMAL BITES

An opossum took up residence in our backyard for a while, and doctors warned me to keep a considerable distance while barbecuing. I was also advised to steer clear of the woodchuck that occasionally pitched up as well. These city transplants often have rabies, as do raccoons, bats, and stray dogs. If any of these charming creatures sinks its teeth into your flesh, scrub the bite and get thee to a hospital, pronto. Rabies is fatal if left untreated, and the hallucinations and pain that occur until one reaches that point are exceedingly unpleasant. As for getting the vaccine preventively, well, it's expensive and you'd need to get a booster within days after being exposed, so it may not be worth it. Like everything, it depends. Preventive shots may make sense if you work in animal control or regularly frequent places where rabies is common and good medical attention elusive, such as parts of Africa and Asia. In any event, give wide berth to any toothy animal foaming at the mouth and to nocturnal ones out for a lunchtime stroll.

As for venomous snakes, bites are painful, but you'll likely survive. No more than fifteen of the average six thousand Americans bitten by poisonous snakes each year die. Australia and Sri Lanka have more venomous serpents than we do; still, the percentage of fatalities there is pretty low, too. As always, prevention is best. Keep a distance of several feet if you're not certain a snake is venomous. Don't provoke the reptile by stomping on the ground or poking it. If it chomps on you, go straight to a hospital. Decapitation does lessen the danger, but the severed head of a rattler can still bite. Do not tie a tourniquet around the wound or cut it and try to suck out the poison; that could actually spread the venom. Don't put ice on the wound, either, or drink alcohol. Booze might dull the pain, but it will also thin your blood. Same with aspirin.

SALT IN WOUNDS

Please, please, don't put salt, or tequila and lime, in a wound. Wounds are not shot glasses.

DIARRHEA AND VOMITING

These common nuisances picked up abroad can wreck a vacation or, worse, a pair of pants. Normally, digestive expulsions from a bug or food poisoning resolve themselves after a few hours. Keep off solids and gradually hydrate to test whether your system can hold down liquids. Take a sip (just a tablespoon) of half water, half Gatorade every ten minutes. This is one of the few times in life when drinking Gatorade is actually healthy for you, because it restores sugar and salt. Chewable Pepto-Bismol will actually kill some bacteria, so always have a pack handy. In general, if the condition is getting better, it will continue to, so don't worry too much. If it's getting worse, however, it will also continue to do so. Blood in the stool and a fever are bad signs. Students always ask, "How long before you die from vomit or the runs?" Don't wait to find out. Get to a doctor after twenty-four hours of sitting on or kneeling in front of a toilet.

CLIMATIC AND EARTHLY MENACES

Altitude Sickness

This charming malady occurs when one rises to a high elevation too quickly and hasn't acclimated. I wish there were an easy cure for this, because I spent eight years feeling miserable while researching a book about mountains. The reporting required that I go as high as ten thousand feet, which was pure agony. I may be overly sensitive, but the feeling of having a construction drill inside your head is existential torture. It feels like the worst hangover ever, multiplied by three thousand. You can't sleep, you can't eat, and you're too dizzy to get anything done, or to rest peacefully, for that matter. Sadly, none of the alleged remedies for altitude sickness, such as ginger and garlic, work for me—not even the tea brewed from the leaves of the coca plant, which is not to be confused with cocoa, or cacao; this is coca as in *cocaine*, and you can get the tea legally in Bolivian mountain towns. But maybe they'd work for you.

Heatstroke and Hyperthermia

Heat exhaustion, or sunstroke, is pretty common; you may have experienced the headache, dehydration, and nausea after a long day at the beach or playing sports. Hyperthermia, however, entails excessive exposure to heat that can damage the brain, heart, muscles, and kidneys and even cause a coma. By excessive heat, I mean a body temperature rising to 104 degrees Fahrenheit (40 degrees Celsius) and above. Telltale signs include a racing heart and rapid breathing, confusion, slurred speech, loss of consciousness, unbearable headache, and even delirium. Minutes matter in this medical emergency. Submerge the patient's body in cool water. If there's no bath to sit in, pour water over them. Arrange evacuation to a hospital. Meanwhile, have them slowly sip water or Gatorade every ten minutes. No gulping it down.

Frostbite and Hypothermia

The thing is, you can acclimate to heat and altitude, but not to extreme cold. Hypothermia occurs when the body temperature drops to 95 degrees Fahrenheit (35 degrees

Celsius) or below. Signs of hypothermia are "mumbles and tumbles"—that is, loss of coordination and concentration, slurred speech, and even passing out. The pulse slows down and breathing becomes shallow.

As for frostbite, the skin becomes numb and red, then blue or white, and then blisters to black. Snowboarders, skiers, mountaineers, soldiers, and the homeless face exposure to this risk. You've probably seen photos of Everest climbers whose noses had black, dead tissue, like they'd charred the noggin on a barbecue. At least they were alive to get a new nose. When we lived in Moscow, people clustered in threes on our street drinking vodka and eating ice cream. *Ice cream!* This was at night in thirty-below-freezing temperatures. One morning, a shopkeeper shoveling snow found a frozen corpse.

Cold exposure is not as rare in the States as people might assume. It seems we're getting more polar vortexes these days, and I've heard stories of college students who went out to parties, drank too much, blacked out in the snow, and got hypothermia. So, if you're going outside in the bitter cold, cover up with adequately warm clothing, stay active, and avoid being out for too long in below-freezing temperatures. And don't even think about "alcohol blankets." These mythical drinks so popular with college students make you *feel* warmer, but they actually draw blood away from where it should be, at the body's core, and toward the skin. Alcohol also clouds judgment, so that in the euphoria of prancing drunkenly in the snow, you may not realize your fingers are developing frostbite and could eventually fall off.

Hand and foot warmers like those sold in camping stores, to be inserted into gloves and boots, may provide some comfort, but they won't save you from hypothermia. If you notice the skin growing waxy and numb, don't rub snow on it. Ice harms skin tissue. Rewarm quickly, preferably inside, with warm, not super-hot, water. If you're helping a friend, give the patient extra clothing and warm them with your own body. Try to keep them conscious with conversation, and don't position them in front of a fire or apply a heating pad. They may be so numb that they won't notice if they're getting burned. Get them to drink warm, sugary liquids, but not caffeine or alcohol, which lead to more heat loss.

Smoke Inhalation and Asthma

If you suffer from asthma attacks, obviously think twice about a vacation to the Sahara Desert, or to California during wildfire season. Even if you go to a tropical rain forest, or stay at home, keep the inhaler by your side—especially on an aircraft. This is why: My friend Bill was on assignment in southern Africa, and his plane crashed upon landing and caught fire. He managed to claw himself out of the wreckage alive, barely, but he suffered the mother of all asthma attacks. The smoke was so bad that his air passages constricted, and he thought he was suffocating, which in a sense he was, because he couldn't inhale properly. He couldn't get to a bronchodilator inhaler, which only increased his panic, which only constricted his airways further. Because the plane had gone down in the middle of nowhere, he couldn't call the local equivalent of 911, or any other emergency responder. He just sat there feeling his airways constricting, convinced he was going to die. He didn't, and he got out of there, but the incident was so traumatic that he gasps for breath, *still*, just thinking about it, and for a long time, he avoided flying. Not flying is a big problem when you're a foreign correspondent and have to be in other countries. But it's an issue for tourists and just about everyone else as well. This brings me to my main point: Anticipate a potentially problematic situation and have on hand what you'll need.

Allergies

If you have a life-threatening allergy, always have an EpiPen at the ready. Equally important, show those with you how to use it properly, should you become incapacitated. Most people with allergies know to pack an EpiPen; the biggest risk can come from others around them not knowing how one works. So, if you're going to die, do it in a heroic fashion and not from a peanut allergy, please.

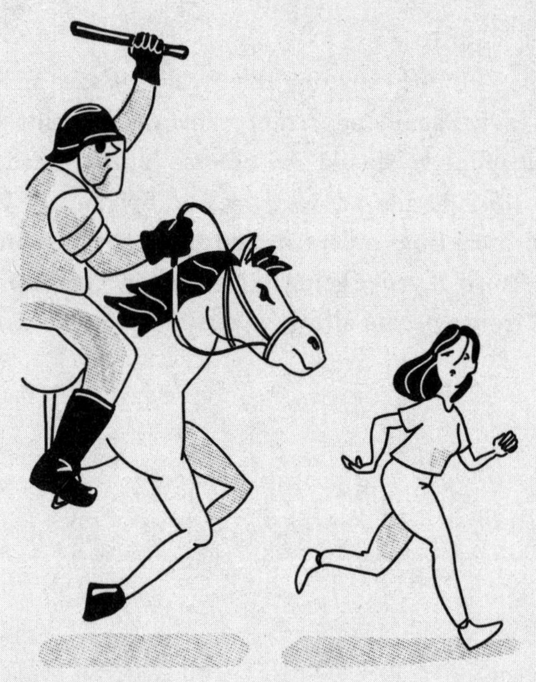

Chapter 5

RUN! PROTESTS, BOMBS, AND SHOOTERS

A French cohort emailed me recently. He's a suave reporter who has covered conventional warfare, assassinations, revolutions, rebellions, militias, ethnic cleansings, coups, attempted coups . . . well, you get the idea. Our paths first crossed in Mexico in 1981, when he was making clandestine contacts with Salvadoran guerrillas. Fifteen years later, I ran into him at a Rwandan church piled ceiling high with skulls. My French friend is one of those professionals who can charm the most riled-up guard at any checkpoint and politely convince a man to put down his machine gun. Now he was confronting barricades of rioting countrymen in his hometown, Paris. He was flabbergasted. This was happening in *Paris*.

Yellow Vest protesters, the formidable *gilets jaunes*, were storming through the city, burning cars and smashing the windows of ritzy boutiques. They took over streets in such numbers that authorities at one point put the city on lockdown and closed the Eiffel Tower and the Louvre. Tourists as well as residents were caught up in the melee. A distant relative of mine who was spending her junior year abroad had gone to the City of Light for a romantic weekend. She chose the wrong weekend. Police rumbling along in armored vehicles blocked the streets, and she choked when they fired ten thousand canisters of tear gas in a vain attempt to disperse the throngs. *Ten thousand canisters*, of a chemical that international law bans for use in war.

Mon ami reported that his neighborhood had not been torched, "yet." But he felt unsafe. His foreign reporting hadn't quite prepared him for unrest at home. He was staying inside as much as possible, but he needed to clear something up for when he next went to the office. He had heard that vinegar served as a barrier to tear gas's toxic effect. (Not true, but more on that later.) Being a French foodie, he had several types in the cupboard and was, in typical chef fashion, weighing the options. "Does balsamic vinegar work as well as white vinegar?" he asked.

I'll answer that question later in the chapter, but the point is that all of us, and not just those headed for war zones, would do well to learn riot defense these days. Let's face it, you could stumble upon a protest skirmish while doing business in Hong Kong or heading to the beach in Puerto Rico. You could attend a different protest in the States nearly every weekend, if so inclined. Left, right, liberal, centrist, war, peace, love, hate—there's a smorgasbord of causes to yell about, and just as many ways to get your point across.

And violent protests can erupt just about anywhere, from Ferguson to Charlottesville to the Arc de Triomphe.

Some people attend demonstrations to have fun and exercise free speech. Others go to kick ass and hurl things. A crowd can turn on a dime, morphing into a chaotic mob in just seconds. Aggression is the chicken pox of protest marches; one minute everyone is all Kumbaya, and then one afflicted individual starts screaming, and the adrenaline kicks in, and the next thing you know, people are whopping each other.

Before you paint the placard and lace up the Ecco boots—essential footwear for demonstrations—do a thorough risk assessment. First, what are the physical and legal risks? (And if you get into a tight spot, whom can you reach out to, and how?) Might you be arrested as well as clobbered on the head? Do you have a criminal record or an outstanding warrant? Will a night in jail impact your career negatively? Are you undocumented, or do you have a medical condition that would complicate detention? Think about how you would be viewed by hostile law enforcement and whether your race or ethnic identity might increase the chance of arrest and harassment. If violence could occur, should you just stay at home? Do you have alternative ways to support the cause and make your voice heard? If so, it's okay to bail, in my book.

VIOLENT PROTESTS

If, after answering all those questions, you still plan to attend a protest, always prepare to be on the receiving end of someone's ire. In a typically volatile protest, which we are seeing with greater frequency in the United States, a certain group shows up with rocks or Molotov cocktails, otherwise known as petrol bombs. These people run amok, setting cars aflame and smashing store windows, or someone's face. If counterprotesters appear, watch out. That could be the start of a brawl. Invariably, the cops storm in, on horseback or in armored vehicles, kitted out in flak jackets and helmets and, in some parts of the world, with snarling dogs and live ammunition. Sometimes the biggest risk is not some riled-up nutcase creating a ruckus but the police tasked with keeping law and order. They add to the confusion by smacking folks on the head or ribs and rounding them up indiscriminately or firing any number of defensive weapons at them. These could include water cannons, sound cannons, tear gas, skunk water, rubber bullets, and real bullets. In the worst-case scenario, folks not only get hurt or unfairly detained, but the poor souls stuck in the middle of the crowd fall to the ground or asphyxiate upright in the crush. At the end of the day, if protesters and innocent bystanders don't end up in the morgue, they can find themselves in the hospital suffering from suffocation, fractures, bruises, abrasions, cuts, or bullet wounds.

Considering how quickly a skirmish can erupt, journalists have cultivated a very sophisticated tactic over the ages to avoid danger: It's called *running.* Failing that, we have a few more tricks in our bags to minimize trouble.

Know What You're In For

First, learn what you might face in order to assess the risks. Reach out to the organizers to find out if they have a permit and a legal team that could bail you out. Generally, it's okay to protest on public property, but not private, although demos in parks or on streets often require a permit from the local authorities. Rules can vary among states and cities. Read news reports about the organizers to ascertain their modus operandi and record of civil disobedience. If you decide to attend a protest, be mentally and sartorially prepared for two days of police custody, and pack essential medication such as insulin, in case you're stuck in jail. Memorize the phone number of your emergency contact and the local chapter of the ACLU and the National Lawyers Guild, in order to seek legal counsel if need be—or write them on your arm in indelible marker. My proxy is my calm husband, who knows how to get ahold of a lawyer on my behalf. Bring enough money for bail, and a driver's license or other form of government-issued identification. And label cameras, phones, and other personal devices with your name in case they are seized.

Snacks are as important as a lawyer in the event of arrest. Protesters can be stuck for hours in a police station or jail without being fed. And once they get food, it's normally some soggy white bread with baloney, which is reason enough to organize an angry protest rally. As a precaution, I always eat a good meal before heading out. Then I make sure to nibble throughout the day, or evening, even if I'm not hungry.

Also, investigate ahead of time what delightful tactical weapon the local police force employs against public assemblies. Ask fellow protesters or organizers and check news reports to see if the cops shoot tear gas or rubber bullets. American police forces across the country embrace diversity . . . of crowd dispersal methods. The downsides of the various tactics vary wildly, from earaches to death. For instance, during the Ferguson, Missouri, turbulence of 2014, the police unleashed smoke bombs, helicopters, flash grenades, rubber bullets, and tear gas to break up crowds. That said, stay abreast of any changes in policing methods. Just to make life difficult, uniformed forces in a given place will often suddenly adopt new approaches if such tactics have made life miserable for protesters elsewhere. During the Occupy Movement of 2011–2012, which spanned about six hundred communities across the United States, protesters had to adapt to an assortment of policing methods as they traveled from city to city. Likewise, familiarize yourself with the type of paraphernalia protesters and counterprotesters usually pack. Concealed firearms? Tiki torches? Baseball bats? Rocks? This sort of information is readily available on the internet. If you plan to attend a protest organized by a particular group, or you hear that counterprotesters intend to show up, review news reports to ascertain their preferred tactics and enemies. Chances are the counterprotesters will not just show up without advance notice.

DRESS FOR SUCCESS

The successful protester chooses diverse accoutrements for different forms of crowd control. Picking the appropriate sartorial accessory is as important as dressing up (or down) the little black dress for the proper occasion. Whether you drape a gas mask over your neck or don ear protectors depends on the event. Consider the following fundamental guidelines as you rummage through your closet:

Wardrobe Neutrality

While I want to intermingle with the crowd, it has to be the right crowd. This means ordinary civilians who do not hurt people. Demonstrations are one of the few times I shun black clothes, in order to avoid being mistaken for a window-smashing anarchist. I'm of the school of thought that one shouldn't be clubbed on the head by neo-Fascists, or police. Any clothes that might make you appear to be a thug or an extremist could make you a target. For that reason, eschew khakis, camouflage, or olive-green garments that send the subliminal message "Weapons!" Camouflage pants or jackets may be the fashion among a certain set, but someone might think you're a provocateur if you wear them, particularly if you're attending protests abroad. Along the same lines, if you're going to a demonstration where everyone is wearing a red MAGA cap, it's provocative to don a pink pussy hat—and vice versa. Oh, and don't cover your face (except to ward off tear gas) or carry big items that look like they could be used as weapons. A bandanna tied around the face is to cops what a red flag is to a bull: It provokes in them an uncontrollable urge to rip it off, slap on handcuffs, and march you to a police wagon.

Comfort

A dress code that signals neutrality proves helpful at protests, as does garb that aids mobility and fleetness of foot. As mentioned before, wear the trusty Ecco boot. Nothing is more pathetic than a limping protester who's lost a sneaker running from counterprotesters. Comfort should reign, too, as protesters are often on their feet longer than anticipated, because they're either having fun or stuck in a thick crowd. Don't put your hair in a ponytail or wear scarves that the police or counterprotesters can use to pull you down. Dangling jewelry can be yanked off. Carry only what you can run with, inside the cross-body bag I recommended in chapter 2 ("The Basics"). Also, check the weather report, and dress in layers and bring water and snacks. You may be on the street or in a damp jail cell for hours more than expected. Sunscreen and rain gear are equally advised, no matter the weather forecast. Along with water and snacks, include toilet paper in your cross-body bag. At some point during a march, everyone has to go, and competing with a hundred thousand protesters for a Starbucks or Porta Potty is challenging enough without the added inconvenience of no toilet paper.

Fisherman Vests

These sleeveless jackets with multiple pockets were all the rage in the 1990s, so much so that Banana Republic stocked them for civilian fashionistas. The many compartments provide ideal storage for essentials: notebooks, pens, phones, memory cards, IDs, credit cards, or anything else you'd want to grab, like lipstick. (If you happen to like trout fishing, it's always worth having a hook or line packed away just in case you stumble upon a riverbank during a melee.) The jackets nor-

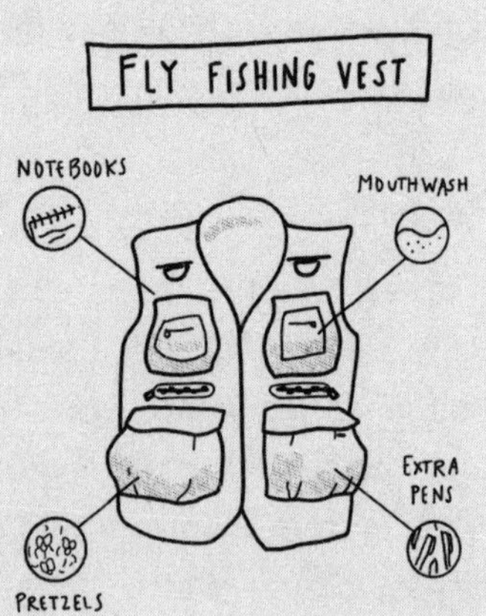

mally come in khaki, but Parisian photographers have been spotted in black versions, and leather no less. This item has gone out of vogue among the correspondent set, which is a darned shame, because it's so handy and can stand in for daypacks. I never was a big fan of giant shoulder pads, but when it comes to the fisherman vest, I'm all for bringing back the 1990s.

Ballistic Helmets

Headgear is awful, too, and not just because of hat hair. It impairs one's ability to take pictures and makes you feel like you have a metal weight on your head. That's because you do. Yet the skull should be protected against flying objects and police batons. You don't need the ballistic variety, unless the police are firing live ammunition. You also may not want to fork out the several hundred dollars it costs to buy one. Bike helmets, construction helmets, and baseball skull catcher's caps all provide varying degrees of protection.

Flak Jackets

Protesters in countries like Venezuela, where the police shoot civilians with live rounds, wear body armor. So far, American police trying to disperse crowds in places like Ferguson and Standing Rock Reservation went only as far as firing the less lethal rubber bullets. But these, too, can cause considerable internal damage upon impact.

Only wear a flak jacket—and ideally, not a navy-blue one—if you absolutely have to. I will go to any length to avoid putting one on because they weigh a ton and, in some cases, make one more of a target. The silhouette they give you will make you resemble SpongeBob SquarePants, even with a loose shirt worn over the jacket. Their weight can vary from fifteen to thirty-five pounds, which makes for uncomfortable wearing, especially in hot weather or if you have to move quickly. A guy at my gym in Manhattan does push-ups in his ballistic vest in order to train. Good for him. But there's no mercy for women with PMS breast soreness. These behemoths are not designed for feminine curves, and they press down on the bosom.

Too often correspondents are handed one and then fall into shock when they actually have to run a mile with the suffocating monster constricting their chest. Breathe deeply, because I have another piece of disturbing knowledge to impart: Once you've been fitted for and have gotten used to lugging this item around on your torso, you shouldn't gain or lose more than 5 to 10 percent of your body weight. If that occurs, you'll have to fork over several hundred dollars for a new vest. So, try to keep the weight stable for roughly five years, as that's the normal lifespan of a flak jacket, if it hasn't suffered too much wear and tear. After that, they are retired—or "condemned," in security industry parlance.

Cameras

Don't lug along tripods or big lenses. They're too hard to run with. I've known photographers to be grabbed by their camera straps and pulled down. One was nearly raped by a mob in India that dragged her to the ground. Photographers who bring several cameras can't run as fast, and as their equipment often takes priority over their personal safety, they can become distracted while protecting their expensive gear from getting smashed. Even a normal-size camera can be hard to hide, so increasingly, photojournalists are using cell phones to document protests; they're easier to put away quickly so you can blend in with the crowd if need be. On the topic of photos, it's legal to take pictures in most public spaces, but not indoors without permission.

KNOW YOUR RIGHTS (AND DON'T ARGUE WITH COPS)

In theory, America embraces robust freedom of expression. The First Amendment enshrines free speech and the right to peaceful assembly. But the police tend to see things differently. Their job is to maintain public order in a situation that can suddenly turn violent or where the people they're supposed to be protecting hate them or wish them harm. Remember: You can't win with cops. They carry firearms and are allowed to use them; you don't and aren't. They have powers of arrest; you don't. They can always justify detention on the grounds that you were disrupting the public peace. If the protest organizers lack a permit, you can be arrested just for being in the vicinity. For that reason alone, nod neutrally if an officer tells you to scram. Keep calm and don't assertively remind him or her of your legal rights—frankly, in such a moment, those rights are irrelevant. I can't tell you how many times protesters or journalists get arrested or beaten for not cooperating. One particular individual who shall remain unnamed often left Occupy Wall Street protests in a police truck, with broken ribs. He never learned. Don't be that guy. Move out of the cops' line of sight if they order you to leave. As soon as their attention shifts to some other poor schmuck, return to whatever you were doing. Oh, and it goes without saying that police brutality is not the time for selfies. In theory, you can take pictures of police, but make sure you can quickly remove and hide the camera's memory card. Cops don't like to be photographed abusing people, and they might detain you on charges of disrupting the peace if you capture their harshness. If you persist regardless, station a friend nearby to grab your iPhone before the cops do.

Most folks who are arrested aren't charged or don't get a criminal record. Generally, protesters only get fined for trespassing or unlawful assembly. But struggling with an officer, obstructing another arrest, failing to disperse, lying in the street, and damaging property will all up the legal ante significantly. If detained, ask to speak to a lawyer. And keep asking, gently, until the officers grant your one free call.

That's in the United States. Free speech looks different in nations that don't have a First Amendment. Many signatories to international treaties ignore this fundamental human right, so I wouldn't set great store by what's on the books. In other parts of the world, opposition gatherings can be banned, or bystanders can be pulled into a dragnet. Trawl news reports to glean how foreign law enforcement deals with protests, and consider whether you might be viewed as a foreign agitator. Carry the number of the nearest U.S. consulate hotline on you, but don't count on American diplomats bailing you out.

Where to Stand

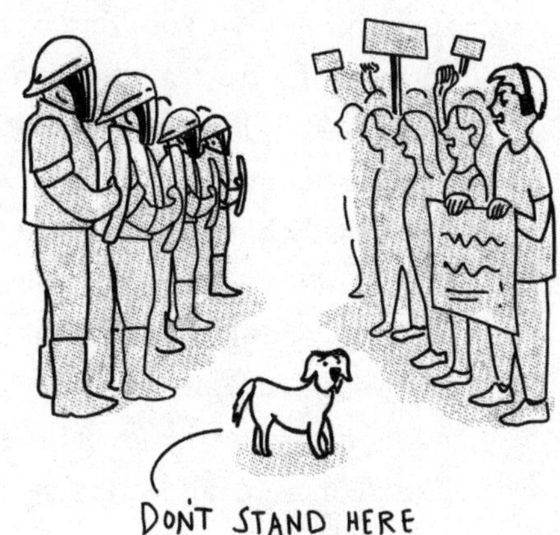

Picture this. There once was a stray dog named Loukanikos, which means "Sausage" in Greek. He was a ginger-colored mongrel who liked to bark at riot police at anti-austerity protests in Athens. Sausage would stand smack in the middle of the protesters hurling petrol bombs and the police shooting tear gas in response. The mutt became an internet sensation, and was mourned around the world when he died in 2014. The cause of death was a heart attack, perhaps hastened by too much tear gas inhalation. While you may crave similar celebrityhood, *do not follow his example*. Do not stand in front of protesters—or police, for that matter. Do not stand at the center of mayhem. Cling to the perimeter of the crowd. This will enable your rapid flight if all hell breaks loose and the crowd stampedes trying to get away.

Don't Argue with Fools

Engaging with aggressive fools will lead to no good. Anger becomes contagious in a crowd. Any protest is one comment away from becoming a riot. Move away before verbal abuse escalates to fisticuffs—or handcuffs.

Plan Your Escape

Have a planned escape route in case your intuition tells you it's time to get out of Dodge. Sense of direction is one of the first things that goes during a panic, and it's not practical to try to figure out where to flee on the fly. Being "height challenged" (read: short), I always fear stampedes because I can't see anything but the torsos around me. Being slight, I can easily be knocked down and trampled. To make up for this handicap, I scope out means of exit ahead of time, and identify landmarks such as tall signs or buildings in order to stay oriented. You can't stop the herd, but you can try to get out of its way and hide behind an object that can't be lifted, like a concrete pillar. Having said that, you don't want to be crushed like an ant against the wall. Choose an object that no one else is running toward.

Most stampede victims die upright, not when they're pushed down or run over. The crowd around them exerts such pressure that they're crushed to death. Imagine a sandwich smushed on both sides so that the filling squeezes all over inside. That's what happens to a body when crushed in a headlong rush of people. The solution? Turn sideways so that your chest is not as exposed and you can breathe. Easier said than done when eight hundred pounds' worth of human beings are pressing against you, but it's essential to survival.

Three's the Charm

In my safety workshops, I ask participants to contemplate a photograph taken at a protest in Athens. A policeman has grabbed a woman's arm, pushing her off balance. A couple of cameras are draped around her neck and she's leaning at a precarious angle in order to protect them. There's no one she can hand them to, or who can negotiate with the cop on her behalf. In such circumstances, she will likely fall, be arrested, have her arm broken, and/or have her memory card seized. A picture's worth a thousand words, as the saying goes, and this photo tells it all: Don't attend protests alone.

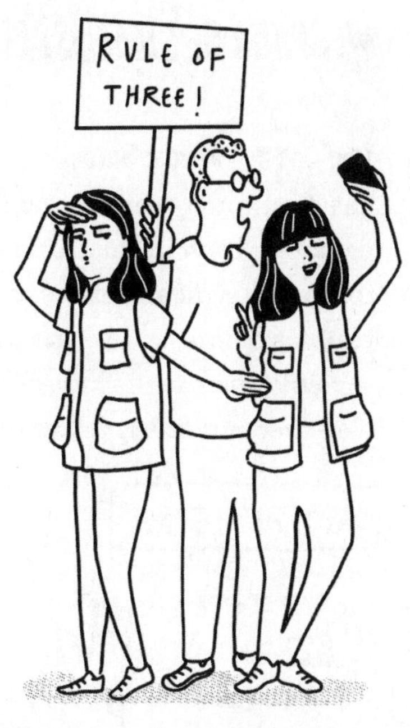

It's more fun to holler slogans with friends, and generally speaking, there's safety in numbers—up to a point. A big group grows unwieldy when trouble strikes. Everyone argues over what direction to flee in, and the next thing you know, you're all the insides of a stampede sandwich, as just described. The ideal is a three-person team—not because of triangles' supposed magical powers but because three makes for efficient teamwork. One person takes pictures of witty placards. Another watches the picture taker's back. The third negotiates with police when they try to grab the other two's cell phones. Extremely tall friends make great companions because they can see over the crowd. While you're at it, write your lawyer's telephone number on the inside of your forearm with water-resistant marker, in case all three of you are arrested. With your wrists handcuffed behind your back, shout your name to strangers standing nearby and ask them to take down the number on your forearm, which will be twisted such that they can copy it. In the best-case scenario, they will call your attorney, whom you warned in advance to expect this call. Aside from the lawyer, the three of you should know how to reach rich friends who can pay bail.

WEAPONS OF SMALL-SCALE DESTRUCTION

Tear Gas and Pepper Spray

The first time I encountered this malevolent tactic, at a demonstration in Guatemala in 1980, I thought I was going to lose my sight and choke to death. I had never encountered tear gas before, so I wasn't prepared for the acrid air. I have sensitive eyes at the best of times, which this wasn't. I doubled over and nearly fell to the ground, gasping. The tear gas made my eyes sting unbearably, and I had trouble seeing and breathing. It didn't help that I was wearing soft contact lenses, which absorbed the irritants and trapped them in my eyes. My skin burned and itched intolerably.

PROTEST GEAR
GLOVES
GOGGLES
DISPOSABLE RAIN GEAR
LIGHTER THAN A REGULAR CAMERA
HELMET
EAR PROTECTORS

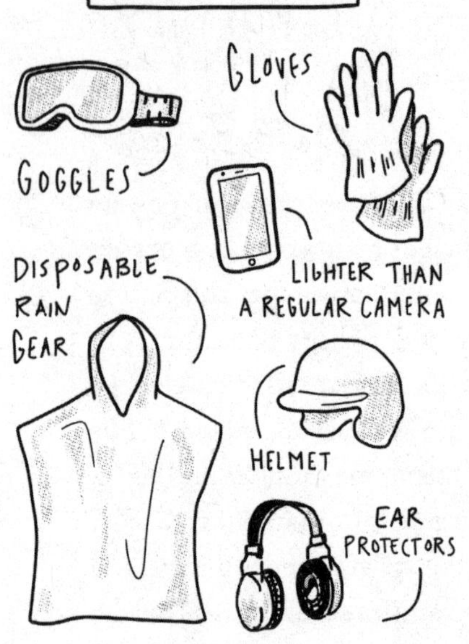

As mentioned earlier, international law bans the use of tear gas in war, but that doesn't stop riot police around the world from deploying this pernicious chemical weapon. It's one of American law enforcement's favorite methods of clearing out protesters, or at least making their day miserable. Most serial protesters have encountered this nasty baby at some point in their demonstrating careers. Contrary to its name, this dispersion tool is not actually a gas but a micro-pulverized powder.

Clouds of these irritating particles are generally meted out with grenade-like canisters. Tear gas doesn't just cause uncontrollable tears. It also sears the lungs and respiratory system. The discomfort can last anywhere from thirty minutes to hours, and even days. You don't build up resistance, and in fact, my doctor believes that my frequent exposure to tear gas may have contributed to my chronic respiratory issues. Certainly in the short-term, exposure to tear gas can worsen the incidence of asthma and bronchitis.

Ask protesters around the world their favorite tear gas remedy, and you'll often hear "vinegar, onion, and lemon." (Hence the query from the French reporter at the start of this chapter.) From Iran to California, protesters tie bandannas rubbed in these cooking ingredients over their noses and mouths, looking like *bandidos* from a bad Western. Urban legend has it that the combination of acids neutralizes the irritants in the tear gas. Bullocks! Whatever acid these foodstuffs contain is insufficient to block the effects of tear gas (although they can be used later to dress a post-protest salad). Also, refrain from "rinsing" the eyes with Coca-Cola, a common practice among Mexican demonstrators. Soda is corrosive and will irritate your eyes. A couple of other key "don'ts": As just indicated, do not wear contact lenses, including hard lenses, which will need to be thrown away. In a similar vein, don't slap on sunscreen, face cream, or makeup when heading out to a protest. Lotions can lock the toxic particles onto your skin. For obvious reasons, mascara is a terrible idea: Not only will your eyes feel like they're burning, but the cosmetic will run in a black stream all over your face.

Disposable rain gear, gloves, and goggles are essential

guards against tear gas. As soon as you leave the scene, throw away items saturated with gas and quickly remove garments and belongings that have been contaminated. Experienced protesters carry an outer layer or change of clothes for this purpose. (The tainted clothes should be washed separately from uncontaminated ones, and for several cycles. Wash them with non-oily soap and cold water as soon as possible.) Only after you've removed the polluted garments should you flush your eyes with a saline solution or cold water. Some protesters carry the rinsing liquid around in a bottle, but bear in mind that just one flush won't work. Water will increase the discomfort at first, but carry on with irrigation; you have to decontaminate, or the tear gas will remain in the eyes. If you wore contact lenses—which, again, is a no-no whenever tear gas might be expected—take them out before flushing the eyes.

The same rinsing regimen goes for the evil cousin of tear gas, pepper spray. When considering a remedy for this skin-scorching substance, think about the digestive tract. One of the best tried-and-true therapies for indigestion is Milk of Magnesia, and this powerful antacid also works wonders for pepper-burned skin. Fill a spray bottle halfway with this chalky white liquid, top it off with water, and apply to affected areas.

If you're going to be exposed to tear gas on a regular basis, consider investing in a gas respirator mask. Upside: It provides the only effective protection against tear gas and toxic fumes. Downside: It can prompt claustrophobia and impedes the wearing of eyeglasses and communication. Just know what you're getting yourself into: You could have a full-blown panic attack when the goggles fog up, you can't see, and you feel like you're trapped in a cage. Swimming or construction goggles might be better suited for the occasion. It's a trade-off. (See Resources.)

Water Cannons

Another charming tactic from the folks in crowd control, and another reason to pack rain gear, is the use of the water cannon. Cannons placed on trucks shoot powerful bursts of liquid to disperse throngs. At its best, the deluge destroys cameras and phones, which is why photographers in particular hate this tactic. (If you anticipate facing the cannon beast, make sure your gear is insured against riot damage.) At its worst, a well-aimed spurt can rupture the spleen. The cannons are particularly effective when the water is mixed with tear gas or pepper spray. Here's a friend's description of a spraying in Panama: "It stung like hell, and because the water soaked your clothes, it was impossible to stop it without stripping and then jumping in the shower." The best protection consists of wearing waterproof clothing, keeping phones and cameras in Ziploc bags, and, better still, sprinting out of range.

Skunk Spray

This putrid monstrosity has to be the most disgusting form of crowd control out there, and I am so glad I've never encountered it. I hope you never do, either. A colleague likened the experience to "being sprayed by runny excrement." Ejected from water cannons, this foul yellow liquid will make everyone in the vicinity sick. It smells far worse than anything sprayed from a skunk, and the stink can fester for days, even weeks. The stench calls to mind sewage or decaying cadavers. It clings to clothes, hair, and skin and permeates everything in its range—buildings, streets, and people who had nothing to do with the demonstration. The Israeli security forces adopted this evil brainchild of a local company about a decade ago and tested it out on Palestinian demonstrators. It's since caught on among militaries and law enforcement agencies around the world. Advocates defend the chemical's use as nontoxic. Protesters on the receiving end, however, complain of nausea, vomiting, retching, respiratory issues, and headaches. No amount of washing will thoroughly remove its traces, so don't wear a favorite sweater if the skunk truck might be heading your way.

Sound Cannons

Sound cannons are also known by the innocuous-sounding name "long-range acoustic devices." Don't be fooled. Portable speakers mounted atop an armored truck blast piercing sounds that can reach up to 150 decibels, well over the level that causes pain and even lasting damage. An acquaintance who got an earful at a protest in Pennsylvania described the attack as "existential" for the level of discomfort caused. Sticking his fingers in his ears didn't make a difference. He toppled over from loss of balance and felt like throwing up. Afterward, he experienced ringing, temporary hearing loss, and sinus pressure. The experience put him off protests for a long time. When he finally ventured out again, he got a good pair of running boots and gun-range ear protectors combined with good earplugs. Pro tip: Bose noise-canceling headphones cannot block a sound cannon's deafening noise.

Kettling

Every time I see a line of police marching toward a large crowd, I move briskly in the opposite direction—especially if they're wielding riot shields or mesh that resembles shrimp nets. Such accessories often mean the law enforcers plan to "kettle" protesters, cordoning them into a contained space. They surround the group and prevent anyone from leaving the site, which raises questions about human rights—such as calling your lawyer or getting medicine in case you faint. Anyone can be swept up, and the cops won't listen to reason if you beg to get away. On the bright side, this crowd-control ploy poses no physical harm, other than causing you to stand for a few hours with a full bladder. Distress increases if you're trapped in the rain without an umbrella, so always pack rain gear just in case.

Horses

I grew up around horses, and never truly feared them until an enormous bay gelding with a policeman on top came charging in my direction at a demonstration. Police use these magnificent beasts for their ability to induce panic. I've never seen a single protester successfully stand ground in front of an incoming steed with a baton-wielding cop riding it. The animals' lethal hooves alone ought to inspire fear. A kick can strike with the force of a small car moving at twenty miles per hour, which means it has the power to smash a skull or cause cardiac arrest. Crumpling into a ball underfoot will not protect vital organs from equine trampling. Horses kick with their hind legs, so don't sneak up from behind one or slap its rump, especially not with an umbrella, as I once saw a protester do.

Rubber Bullets

They sound so pleasant: soft, gentle drops that plop off you. Don't be fooled. These allegedly nonlethal projectiles can most certainly kill if fired directly at an internal organ. More benevolently, they fracture bones and leave horrific bruising. British security forces first deployed these menaces in the 1970s in Northern Ireland, and rubber bullets have caught on among riot police around the world as a popular alternative to real ones. It can take weeks to mend if you get hit, and some victims never fully recover, physically or emotionally. Your best defense is to duck or get away fast.

Pellet Guns

A common form of crowd control against stone-throwing protesters in Kashmir, the pellet gun, or pump-action shotgun, can blind and even kill. Numerous Kashmiris have lost their sight after being hit. Due to the pellet gun's efficacy in scattering demonstrators, I wouldn't be surprised if a police force near you begins to assemble an arsenal. Take the same defensive action as with rubber bullets: Stay low, take cover, and run!

Tasers

Also known as stun guns, these weapons have high currents that are meant to incapacitate. Two barbed darts shoot out, and upon contact cause skeletal muscles to freeze by overriding the central nervous system. Generally, the biggest risks from tasers for a healthy person are falling and bruising; the pain and loss of control of one's movements will eventually subside. However, people have suffered cardiac arrest following shocks. I don't recommend sticking around to find out if you're one of those people!

ACTIVE SHOOTERS

I sometimes teach high school students, and my heart breaks at the number who have been exposed to mass shootings in their communities. They continue to be haunted by massacres at their schools years after the events—and that's just the kids. Some adults have lived through more than one incident, too. I recently heard from a woman in Southern California who has experienced not just one active shooter situation but three. *Three.* The violence is getting out of hand, and I find myself increasingly geared up just in case. Only the other day, my husband and I were driving on the highway toward Las Vegas and a road sign flashed that two dangerous convicts had escaped prison in a red vehicle. Naturally, we immediately watched for cars that matched that description and prepared to drop to the floor if one drove past with a gun barrel sticking out the window. When we pulled into a rest stop to fill up, my peripheral vision went into full gear, and I got ready to crouch by our car's wheel should the escapees join us in the parking lot. I calculated how fast I could dash to hide in the women's room. (Ten seconds? Hopefully.)

Whether or not a gunman sprays bullets from a vehicle or storms into a movie theater, some general principles can help you survive the crisis—namely, stay calm, stay low, and get off the X (military parlance for crosshairs). Chapter 12 gives guidance on how to maintain your cool to avoid freezing up; after all, you need to function on all cylinders. If you can't run, take cover. Most mass shootings last just a few minutes, so they're often over before authorities arrive to save the day. That means you have to stay laser focused.

Concentrate on figuring out where the shooting is coming from and getting out of the line of fire. The loudness of the noise should indicate the shooter's proximity. Make an emergency call if you can and then turn all your attention to survival.

Fleeing should be the first plan of action. With gunfire, unlike protests, being short presents an advantage, as it's more difficult to hit a smaller target. That should not instill complacency, however. Lots of variables determine whether a shooter will hit a bull's-eye, including his training, the type of weapon, and his distance from targets. A Navy SEAL sniper can hit the bull's-eye from nearly a mile away, but the average Joe with a handgun will probably miss most of his targets. That goes for well-trained cops, too. According to one study, the hit rate in gunfights for officers in the NYPD was only 18 percent. (See Resources.) However, the AR-15 rifle favored by mass shooters has a high kill rate because it spews out vast numbers of high-velocity bullets that savagely tear flesh upon impact. The Las Vegas shooter, who murdered fifty-eight people in October 2017, fired hundreds of rounds from an automatic rifle within minutes, from more than one thousand feet away. Make yourself less of a target by bending over and running in a zigzag pattern, at a diagonal from the gunman's position.

Unfortunately, this is much harder than it sounds, especially for those of us with bad knees. Practice doesn't necessarily make perfect, but it helps. Try it in a neighborhood park or street, if you can stand all the strange looks you'll get. You might even make new friends! I tried this move once in Central Park, and some intrigued onlookers thought it was a new fad and zigzagged behind. Taking into consideration the chances of someone's being hit, even if they're bent over and running in this awkward position, learn basic first aid (consult chapter 4), such as applying tourniquets and pressure to wounds so the victims around you don't bleed out.

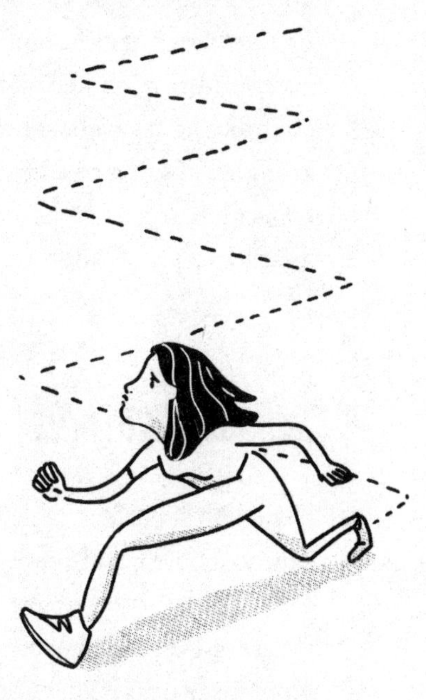

Taking Cover

If you can, run inside or behind something big and sturdy, like a wall, a building, or a dumpster. Bullets can pass through almost anything, but an object will slow the shooter down and obscure his line of fire. Avoid windows, as shattered glass could cut you. Cinder block disintegrates into fragments when hit by bullets, and the dust gets into lungs and eyes and can become embedded in skin. Buildings all over the world are made with cinder block, but a cinder block building is a risk worth taking if it's the only option. As for cars: Forget Hollywood. Bullets can pierce cars. Cowering behind a vehicle will save you only if you pick the right part: The wheels and engine block can serve as barriers, to some extent. In any case, duck behind whatever you can, and if you're able to, turn a corner. Whether you stay put or move depends on whether the firing is far away. Don't pop up like a prairie dog to see if the killer's gone. Stay low (like knee high) when trying to catch a glimpse from behind your barrier. I always suggest my trainees get accustomed to the noise of incoming versus outgoing fire by watching

YouTube videos of various weapons being shot. The source of the bangs and booms will depend on the situation and surroundings, as aerodynamics plays a role in what a shot sounds like (as well as how a bullet travels). You'll get a general idea of what to expect, but as a rule, a handgun will not be as loud as a high-velocity assault rifle; the latter produces a rapid series of bangs.

SCHOOL SHOOTINGS

Sheltering in Place

Many schools and workplaces have protocols for where to hide and how to behave if you're trapped inside a building where a gunman is roaming around in the corridors. Ask your institution for guidelines for what to do in the event of a lockdown. If it has no protocol, initiate a discussion on creating one. If it holds drills and they are upsetting psychologically, have a frank discussion about the impact. Chapter 12 discusses how to deal with the emotional fallout from such a traumatic event. Typically, a lockdown will involve emptying the hallways; covering the windows of the room you're in, so no one can look in; pushing furniture against the doors; moving everyone away from the windows and doors; locking doors; sitting on floors; and turning off lights. Those who hide in bathrooms should crouch on the toilet seats with their heads down so that the shooter can't spot legs or heads. Do not make noise while hiding. Debates rage over whether one should throw objects at an attacker, or even keep cell phones switched on. Obviously, one wants to text for help and stay in touch with loved ones, but any sound could give away hiding spots or positions. At the very least, mute your phone's ring and other sound notifications so as not to draw attention to yourself.

As for fighting back, don't do anything that might aggravate the situation. You could hurl a chair at the attacker if you have no other option than to die; it's worth a try if you can help those nearby in the process and shift the gunman off his course. However, the gunman's course is a hard thing to establish in the volatile moment, and a well-armed person with a semiautomatic weapon will probably keep shooting regardless.

DRESS FOR SUCCESS

Bulletproof Backpacks

I get a fair number of queries from parents about bullet-resistant backpacks, meant to keep students safe in the event of a school shooting. I completely understand that impulse: I, too, want to make sure I am doing everything possible to protect my own son. It's terrifying to send your kid to school these days, knowing how many have been shot in their classrooms; it's an appalling thought. But save your money: Don't get one of these backpacks. It's not worth buying the kids an expensive bag that most likely will not be on them at the time of a shooting or provide adequate protection.

As with flak jackets, the effectiveness of these backpacks expires after five years, and they shield the wearer only against handguns. The Kevlar plates are considered "soft" body armor, and thus are useless against the semiautomatic rifles (like the AR-15) favored by mass shooters.

Most important, students don't usually have their backpacks on them at all times. Once they take out the books they need, they generally leave the bags in their lockers. In any case, the weight of the backpacks alone will discourage students from lugging them around from room to room, and extended wearing could cause injuries. If you do press ahead, ensure that the model you choose is certified by the National Institute of Justice, the R&D arm of the Department of Justice. This organization's stamp of approval guarantees quality.

BOMBS

"If you see something, say something," the government slogan goes. Yet most of us don't have that highly tuned eye to judge whether the sweating, pacing man on the train platform is about to detonate a suicide vest or is simply late to a meeting. Likewise, does that gym bag sitting with trash on the curb contain an explosive device, or did someone throw it out because the zipper broke? These security quandaries can drive a good citizen crazy, particularly somewhere like New York City, where everyone dumps junk on the sidewalk—old appliances, dirty clothing, and mattresses infested with bed bugs. Author-

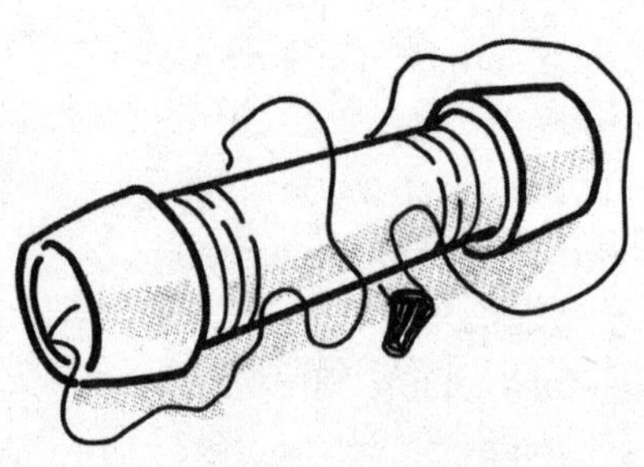

ities have received thousands of calls about suspicious packages since 2001, but most (thankfully) have turned out to be false alarms.

That said, trust your gut if something seems off, such as smoke curling from a parked car in Times Square. Two street vendors did just that in May 2010, and foiled a terrorist plot in the heart of New York City. Even if there hadn't been a bomb ticking inside the vehicle, smoke pluming from parked cars should always be reported, as a general rule.

A common explosive device made in America is the pipe bomb. As the man who sent some to critics of President Donald Trump in 2018 discovered, they are easily assembled with everyday components such as PVC pipes, nails, screws, bolts, fireworks, electrical wire, and cell phones; likewise, pressure cooker bombs like the ones detonated by the Boston Marathon bombers. So, be ready to call 911 if you're in a hardware shop and a twitchy customer asks for all these items, or you happen to see a pipe lying on the sidewalk with wires sticking out of it. Same with a suspicious-looking package that arrives in the mail. Do not try to disassemble it yourself or nudge it with your toe. A fellow writer in Spain opened a letter bomb from a disgruntled reader and lost part of his fingers and some hearing. Leave the detonation to authorities and get away fast.

Even if you don't see one of these contraptions lying around, it doesn't hurt to identify exits anytime you're near a locale that might be a target, such as a shopping mall, bridge, government building, transportation hub, theater, hotel, sports venue, school, concert hall, or house of worship. In other words, nearly everywhere. Let's throw in amusement park as well—not that I'm whipping up panic here . . .

To inflict maximum casualties, sometimes terrorists will detonate a second bomb when emergency responders arrive in response to the first explosion. Unless you require immediate medical attention, run at least a few blocks away from the bomb site, steering clear of any unattended vehicles and buildings that have been hit. The former might contain explosives, and the latter could rain down shattered glass and debris.

Stay Calm

Like it or not, the bottom line is that situations involving terrorist attacks and active shooters are not within your control. Your best bet is to stay calm. Not easy, of course, but try to keep cool. Take deep breaths, pray if you believe in God, and if not, tell yourself that this will pass. It will eventually, and hopefully you'll survive intact. Hopefully, too, you've done your research and prepared mentally. That's the best you can do.

Chapter 6

DO I STAY OR DO I GO? NATURAL DISASTERS

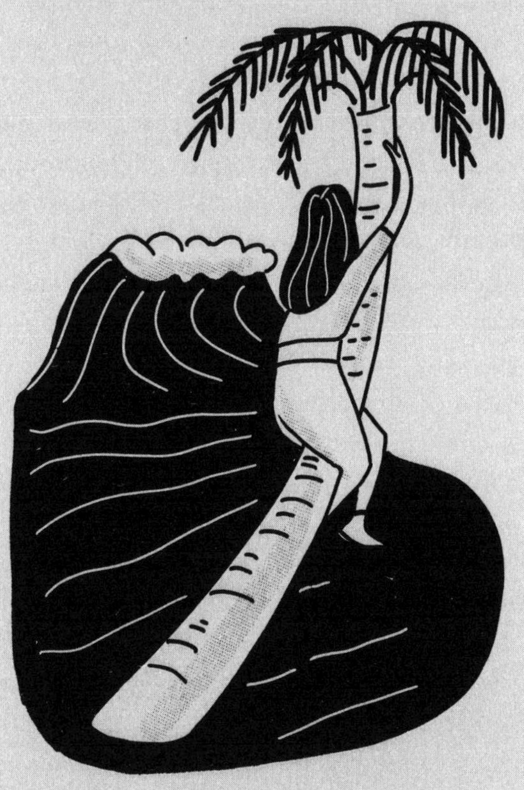

Whether or not you believe in climate change, Mother Nature doesn't care. She just does what she does. And she's been truly vicious lately, unleashing disasters of spiraling frequency and force. The United States' being a huge and geographically diverse country, no corner is safe from natural catastrophe. Americans all over the land can face, variously, earthquakes, volcanoes, drought, Arctic chill, hurricanes, tornadoes, lightning, wildfires, wind, and floods—or a combination thereof. Between 2000 and 2019, environmental calamities killed more than ten thousand Americans, and damages topped $1.6 trillion. The year 2017 was the worst on record, with fourteen weather "events" that caused losses of $306 billion. (See Resources.) The global toll is uncountable. Scientists say this is our new normal, and the new normal particularly kills women. According to the World Bank, women are much more likely than men to die in natural disasters, because women tend to be less mobile when severe weather hits. Being pregnant or homebound, or caring for elderly parents or children, slows us down from getting in the car and out of town. After Hurricane Katrina, most of the victims trapped in New Orleans were women and children. Pregnant or nursing mothers face additional challenges. A lack of potable water and medical care, infectious diseases, and the stress of running from a collapsing building or witnessing a death all increase the risk of maternal or infant mortality. Hospitals may run out of supplies or be hard to reach due to wrecked or flooded roads. Breastfeeding will be interrupted if the infant is ferried far from the mother, as happened after Katrina. As if that weren't bad enough, some women will avoid going to evacuation shelters for fear of being raped, a not-unreasonable fear as domestic violence and sexual assault flare during disasters.

So, how do you get ready for these natural emergencies? While no one-size-fits-all dominates, certain principles dictate planning for any natural disaster, be it a spewing volcano or a typhoon. These are: (1) knowledge of local weather and climatic patterns; (2) a communication plan to remain in contact with authorities and loved ones; (3) an escape plan; and (4) an emergency kit (see page 140).

I suggest preparing as though for an outlandish and never-ending camping trip, because that's pretty much what it can come to—an excursion where everyone gets the runs, a tree falls on your head, and a thunderstorm downs power lines so you can't call for help or watch Netflix. Every disaster is different, but my friend Tina, whom you met in the chapter on first aid (chapter 4), swears by three essentials: cash, electronic communications, and clean underwear. She says these saw her through many hurricanes, earthquakes, and at least one tsunami. The cash bought food and a place to sleep; the devices ensured a way to stay in touch with emergency updates and loved ones; and the clean underwear made her feel at least somewhat refreshed each day, no matter how filthy her surroundings. ("And undies take up practically no space in a bag," she notes. "Pack 'em all!")

As for planning, Tina shared her approach with hurricanes, which have a particularly long emergency period, one that lasts before and after the actual disaster hits. Businesses tend to shut their doors forty-eight hours or so before predicted landfall, gas stations run out of fuel as everyone tries to flee, and the power usually goes out for days, meaning gas pumps and ATMs won't be working. Tina's first hurricane was Ivan, in 2004, which made landfall as a "strong category 3" storm in Florida and Alabama. She managed to score a room at a Mobile hotel before the predicted landfall. (Note: Hotel rooms sell out quickly during a disaster, so move fast at the first hints of trouble. You can always cancel the reservation if the winds change.) She rented a high-clearance SUV. (This is another good tip for disasters—you can sleep in it quite comfortably if there are no hotels, but not in heavy floods, of course.) The day before the storm hit, she made a point of stopping at every open gas station to fill up, as it was clear the gas pumps were going to start running dry, and she wanted as much fuel as possible for when disaster struck. She also figured the power would be out for several days, and the hotel kitchen wouldn't be functioning, so she stopped at an open supermarket and stocked up on nonperishables: sardines and tuna (with pop-top cans, not the kind that require a can opener) and a bottle of red wine (screw top, of course). Then she spotted one of the few "restaurants" still open—a Subway sandwich shop. She swung through and ordered five foot-long Veggie Delite Subs with extra mustard but no mayo, to see her through the powerless, nonrefrigerated days in her future. She kept them lined up on the counter in front of the TV and looked forward to eating half of one each day for lunch and another half each night for dinner, along with some of that wine. And she didn't forget dessert! Seeing an open McDonald's, she snapped up ten little apple pies (which were also great for breakfast). "No idea what they're made of, but they don't spoil and actually taste good, even after sitting in a paper bag for days," Tina says.

When Ivan made landfall, she lacked electricity for at least four days, but had enough gas to get far away if necessary. She made contact with the office and stayed abreast of emergency updates from the car using the 12-volt adapter she always carried, ate apple pie for breakfast, and rationed the rest of the food for the remainder of her stay. When she left, she donated unopened sardines and tuna to a Red Cross shelter.

In this case, Tina stayed put because her job demanded that. As you figure out whether to flee a location, I suggest appointing yourself as the household member to handle emergency preparations, as self-reliance creates more self-confidence. I've found that in many relationships, one person does the shopping lists and kids' schedules, and the other pays the bills and changes light bulbs. It's rarely "Let's do it all together." So, I would say the grocery store shopper is probably well suited for the disaster kit task. I particularly like this role because it gives me a sense of control in a terrifying situation. Plus, there's nothing like being in charge and bossing other people around.

Now that we've established that you're running the show, here's what you need to do:

KNOWLEDGE IS POWER

Familiarize yourself with the local climatic conditions and geology that might cause a crisis, as well as warning signs that calamity is approaching. (A number of disasters can create a thunderous roar, among them tsunamis, avalanches, tornadoes, and landslides. By the time you hear them, though, it's probably too late to get out of their path.) Obviously, Tornado Alley lies in the Great Plains, and the Pacific Northwest is tsunami/earthquake territory. Hurricanes occur late in the summer, and wildfires whenever it's hot and dry. But once you've established that you don't live in an area prone to tornadoes or whatever, consider all the freaky climatic stuff that is going on these days, which may take authorities, and you, by surprise. For instance, Brooklyn experienced a twister a few years back. Brooklyn! It wasn't quite *Wizard of Oz* level, but it blew off some roofs and wrecked a hundred cars. Bad events often have a domino effect, so your worst-case scenario is going to include the potential for more than one event, such as a tandem tsunami and earthquake, or floods following cyclones. Hills denuded by wildfires produce mudslides. Volcanoes can trigger earthquakes. You get the picture. You've gotta be prepared for a lot of bad events.

COMMUNICATIONS

On the off chance you've discovered that, say, a devastating tropical storm could head your way, sign up for early alerts with local authorities and ask them about evacuation routes and emergency contact numbers. Does the city sound alert sirens? Tune into local radio stations for updates. (You can't necessarily rely on text alerts. I'll get to that later on.) Buy a hand-cranked radio with a USB charger for smartphones and emergency beacons and alerts that are color-coded. The crank powers up the radio's internal battery, so you won't need batteries! A device labeled "NOAA Weather Radio" will receive updates during emergencies from the National Weather Service. You will appreciate the news stories advising when you can reemerge into the world.

Store emergency contact info on a piece of paper as well as your cell phone, which will of course remain juiced up nonstop, with a spare battery on hand, before and during the crisis. Text and Twitter prove vital for receiving alerts and updates, so rely on smartphones rather than landlines. (This is for the seven people in the world who still have the latter.) There's always the possibility that the cell network will crash, which is another reason you'll want a hand-cranked radio on hand for emergency updates. In order to streamline messaging, set up a group list that includes all the people you'd want to reach—kids' teachers, coworkers, family, babysitters, friends. Contacts should include an out-of-towner, as it's often easier to reach someone outside a disaster zone. (That happened to me during September 11, 2001. My husband and I couldn't communicate with each other on Manhattan island, but my mother managed to make calls to each of us from an outer borough.) While you're at it, make sure the younger kids know your telephone number in case of separation. Have them memorize it with a song or chant: "Six-four-six, we're in a fix / Nine-two-five, we're still alive / Nine-one-three-four, we're out the door!"

Lack of communication is one of the most unsettling aspects of disasters, and being able to call for help is critical. Consider buying, or renting, a satellite telephone. Ships use them when far from terrestrial mobile phone sites, and they work on land, too. I used to take such an apparatus everywhere that was remote and ruined, which was essentially everyplace I worked. They connect to orbiting satellites, so you can telephone from jungles and deserts when you're out of cell range, and they're de rigueur during tsunamis and other calamities when cell towers fail. Satellite phones were a lifesaver for acquaintances in Puerto Rico when the devastating hurricane hit, and reporters found them invaluable during Katrina. "Sat phones," in emergency parlance, have come a long way from when I first used them in the 1990s. Back then, the devices measured the size of a coffee table and required half an hour to assemble. Models today resemble laptops or a bulky cell phone from the 1980s. Used ones sell for about five hundred dollars. Calls per minute cost a fortune, but it's worth the price if this is your only means of staying in touch with the outside world.

While you're at it, invest in a surge protector. As mentioned earlier, I once blew up an old-style sat phone that cost ten thousand dollars (thankfully, not of my money) because I didn't realize that power spikes when it comes back on after a blackout. (It does, big time, and my boss was not pleased.) Surge protectors are super for any emergency that might blow a transformer, even a powerful thunderstorm. These items don't last forever, though, so get a replacement once yours has been used in an emergency. I learned that lesson the hard way, too.

GET OUT OF DODGE

If officials say evacuate, then *go*. Don't be one of those people who refuse to leave their homes in a category 5 hurricane and then waste valuable resources being rescued. That puts a strain on emergency responders who should be saving the lives of sick or elderly folks who truly couldn't get out, as opposed to stubborn individuals who chose to remain. To find a shelter closest to you in the event that authorities call for an evacuation, text SHELTER plus your ZIP code to 43362 (4FEMA). So, if your zip code is 10021, you would text SHELTER 10021.

Just for the hell of it, I recently checked whether New York still had fallout shelters, as I see the markings all over the city. It turns out that the thousands of shelters designated during the Cold War are no longer active, as that threat has long passed and the city has no plans to revive them. During our last big hurricane, Sandy, the city selected schools all over town as shelters. One lies a convenient three blocks from my house; another, six streets away. Failing that, my building has a basement and several rooms to hide in. Once you've figured out where to go, discuss this evacuation plan with your family and the kids' school, as well as where to go in case you can't contact one another or not everyone can reach that spot. If you think you might want to skedaddle out of town entirely, check with cousin Lucy beforehand and confirm that you can crash at her house (and ascertain that Fluffy the cat is truly welcome). Courtesy goes a long way when you're camping in someone's living room for four months.

Apropos, many hotels and shelters won't accept animals. Confirm ahead so that you and Rover aren't stranded when the floodwaters rise. Make sure the pet's collar has your name and number attached, in case of separation. And pack paraphernalia such as the pet's bowl, leash, litter, food, water, medications, vaccination cards, and carrier. Plan on two weeks of supplies.

Finally, do a test run of the emergency evacuation. As for a wedding, rehearsals will make you feel more confident when the big day arrives. Ready the getaway car well before an emergency, in order to avoid scrambling at the last minute. Fill the gas tank to the brim, put air in the tires, and pack spares. Park the car in a garage or driveway facing out, to enable a swift exit. (Journalists do this routinely, to save time in case of an urgent story, not just when the weather portends disaster.) Get into the habit of sleeping with clothes and shoes near the bed. (War correspondents will often sleep with their boots on in case of a sneak attack, but that's not the optimal way to get a sound night of Zs.)

Oh, and before leaving the house, turn off the gas and unplug electrical appliances and other items (including the fridge, which you regularly defrost, right?). You don't want them to catch fire and then return to a burned-down abode.

EMERGENCY KIT

Think of the emergency kit as a ready-to-go bag on steroids. It has more supplies, which are geared toward survival rather than simply layering for the right climate. For insurance purposes, take an inventory of the house before the catastrophic event—like *now*. Photograph possessions and the interior and exterior of Home, Sweet Home. Make copies of all valuable documents and store them in a waterproof pouch. By valuable, I mean identification, passports, insurance policies, doctors' contacts, medical records if someone in the family has a serious preexisting condition or is pregnant, photos and immunization records of pets (in case they get separated), immunization records for the human family, birth and marriage certificates, bank statements, home insurance/deeds, and voter registration cards.

Some earthquake experts suggest packing an emergency kit for the car, home, *and* office, as you never know where you'll be when the Big One wallops. Regardless of what you choose, essential items for the car include beacons, flares, a shovel, a fire extinguisher, jumper cables, maps—you can't rely on GPS when the system crashes—spare tires, a jack, and spare gasoline.

Your all-purpose emergency kit will have the extra cash that Tina mentioned, spare house keys, an emergency blanket, lighters and waterproof matches, and a beacon. A whistle comes in handy if you get trapped, as does a multipurpose tool that includes a knife, a file, pliers, a screwdriver, a can opener, and preferably a corkscrew. Also, an LED flashlight. I like the headlamp variety that shines from the forehead. It frees the hands to do things like apply bandages and dig out the car. Your three days of supplies should include nonperishable food, water, utensils, a can/bottle opener, toiletries (soap, wipes, toothbrush/paste, shampoo, deodorant, feminine hygiene products), diapers and baby formula for little ones, spare eyeglasses, towels, and a change of clothes. And of course you've remembered the medical kit from chapter 2.

The following are the most common health issues that arise during or after various natural disasters:

- Panic, depression, abrasions, fractures, bruises, cuts, gastro and respiratory issues, infections;
- Burns (wildfires, volcanoes, chemical/radiation accidents, and electrical fires in the event of earthquake);
- Heart attack, drowning, and asphyxiation (nothing in a medical kit can help—sorry); and
- Gunshot wounds from scenes of looting.

Last, always pack hope. It doesn't fit in the kit, but it's often a lifesaver.

DRESS FOR SUCCESS

Heat

More than nine thousand Americans have died from heat-related causes since 1979. Heatstroke is among the leading causes of death in young adults and teens. It can pose terrible health risks when the air-conditioning fails in power outages. Wear lightweight, light-colored, loose-fitting fabrics that wick moisture. They allow the skin to breathe and perspiration to evaporate and cool the body. Long trousers and sleeves protect skin from exposure. Carry an umbrella or put on a wide-brimmed hat, preferably with vents and of a breathable material. These will prevent the sun from warming the head. You also need to hydrate and stay in the shade.

Wildfires

Wildfires call for nonsynthetic materials, such as leather boots and wool or cotton, that won't melt onto your skin if they catch alight. Fire usually kills by damaging the lungs and asphyxiation, so consider keeping respirator masks in the house and car. The N95 construction model is fine for heavy dust particles or pollution à la China, but one should don something more durable for smoke and burning chemicals. Home Depot sells a variety that painters use to guard against fumes. You'll look like an ant monster from a sci-fi movie, and perhaps get claustrophobic wearing the mask, but fires are not a time to worry about such things.

The Polar Opposite—Polar Vortex

During that bone-chilling week in January 2019 when below-freezing temperatures affected 140 million Americans, killing nearly a dozen, I was prepared. Living in Russia had left me with a formidable armoire of warm layers. On went the thermal leggings, merino undershirt, turtleneck pullover, wool, fleece, cashmere socks, cashmere shawl, boots, puffy hooded coat, and ski gloves. (Note the repeated mention of cashmere. I learned to appreciate its warmth in the Himalayas, where the Kashmiri goat lives. The soft fiber lends a luxurious feel while you waddle around like the Michelin Man.) I topped it all off with a mink hat. Yes, fur. When I moved to Moscow, my mother gifted me a mink hat from a thrift shop. Minks sleep in the snow. They stroll in blizzards. They can handle a Siberian, or Minnesotan, wind chill of minus-fifty degrees. I understand if dressing in dead mammals upsets you. Our family had a pet chinchilla, so no one will ever persuade me to wear his cousins. But I have no problems with mink, or shearling, because those creatures never lived in my house. Their pelts keep you massively toasty and look glamorous besides. However, I get that vegetarians find that disgusting, and I buy only animal garments that are secondhand. For

PETA-certified items with style, order brands from Quebec. French-speaking Canadians have perfected *la mode* for winter so that they don't look like fat ducks in clumping boots. Whatever your fabric choice, sunglasses and goggles with 99 percent UV block are nonnegotiable, to protect against snow blindness. This damaging and painful condition is in effect a sunburned eye. The affliction occurs when UV rays reflect off snow and ice, especially at a high elevation. People who have had laser corneal surgery are particularly vulnerable to the severe drying from cold weather, so they may want to ignore my earlier advice about the operation ("Eyeglasses versus Surgery") in chapter 2.

Before I forget, keep handkerchiefs handy. These don't really qualify as clothing, but they're just as important as the right coat. When I lived in the former Soviet Union, they saved me from great embarrassment. You see, in frigid cold, snot freezes in the nose. Then, after you've been inside awhile, the mucus defrosts in a gush. It always seemed to happen to me at a party or during an important interview. Generally, one senses that the dam is about to open, so there's enough time to grab the hankie.

Hurricanes

Melania Trump wisely changed out of stilettos before inspecting damage from Hurricane Harvey. No one, not even the president's wife, should teeter on skyscraper poles in such circumstances. Heels are for galas, not disaster sites where victims drown. When it comes to hurricanes, not even the mighty Eccos will do. Extreme times call for extreme measures. Go all out with knee-high rubber boots.

WHEN THE POWER GOES OUT

Perishables can stay fresh for about twelve hours if you keep the fridge door closed. Move them to the freezer section for an even longer shelf life. After a day, throw away medication that requires refrigeration. Generators should be set up twenty feet from the house, to avoid carbon monoxide poisoning. Water purification systems may fail when the power goes, so don't take chances with tap water. Drink bottled instead.

Stay inside the car if a power line falls on it. If the vehicle then catches fire, leap out as far as you can and maintain a distance of at least fifty feet.

AS TOLSTOY SAID

The emergency kit and general strategies I've outlined will see you through most anything. However, to paraphrase Tolstoy's quote that "every unhappy family is unhappy in its own way," each calamity has its own miserable peculiarities. Even though we have little (read: zero) control over Mother Nature's whims, it's helpful to know what you're up against. And if you live in or are traveling to an area that's prone to a particular disaster, you'll want to spend extra time and attention preparing for the complications that can arise.

Hurricanes, Typhoons, and Cyclones

They're all different names for the same thing: torrential rains with heavy winds that occur in summer months. All cause equal destruction. Aside from having your roof blown off or your car swept away, the biggest problems come with not evacuating when told to and failing to find high ground above the ensuing floodwaters. The aftermath can be more dangerous than the actual storm, as sewage leaks into the water supply, bringing bacteria and disease. You'll know a weather system is approaching by watching television newscasters stand in torrential rains with their hair blowing in the wind. Drops in barometric pressure, severe headaches, and swells on the sea's surface portend that it ain't gonna be pretty.

I've heard people advise seeking shelter in a basement or cellar. This makes sense for tornadoes but not massive rainstorms. While heading underground provides protection against gales, the accompanying water can cause several feet of flooding. If you have any inclination to go into the cellar during the next big hurricane, pull up some old photos of Katrina, during which desperate people sought help on their roofs. While the storm is raging, seek shelter in an interior room without windows, like a bathroom, or in a closet. Make yourself comfortable under a sturdy table in case the roof collapses. After the winds die down, move up to higher floors, even the creepy attic.

As for preparation at the onset of storm season, trim branches that hang over the house and move the grill and the potted plants inside. Keep gutters and pipes clean. I learned the hard way that drains clogged with debris can bring on basement floods that cause thousands of dollars of repairs not covered by house insurance. Tie down anything that might float away, and lock and board up windows with heavy plywood. Urban legend has it that taping windowpanes with duct tape in the shape of an X will buttress the glass from shattering. Not true. Get plywood.

Tornadoes

Devilishly twisting columns of air comprise one of the most destructive weather systems on earth. The United States reports more than 1,200 tornadoes annually, generally east of the Rockies. Tornado season falls in spring or summer, depending on the location. Telltale signs include a rotating, funnel-shaped cloud, churning debris, and a loud roar resembling a train. Take cover immediately if you spot a girl with braids and a small dog in a basket being carried away. Flying debris presents the biggest danger. Avoid windows, doors, and outside walls. Rush into a strong building and down to the basement or into an interior room on the lowest level, or a closet, away from windows. If outdoors, do not seek protection under bridges or overpasses. These figure among the worst places to be because winds of up to two hundred miles per hour can channel debris underneath them. If inside a car, pull over (though not under an overpass), strap on the safety belt, and cradle your head. That said, tornadoes can flip over vehicles, but it's better than standing in a cornfield.

Wildfires

If you live in a drought-prone place with lots of dry wood and power lines that easily catch fire (read: California), prepare the emergency kit today and sign up for alerts from local authorities. The minute that ominous text arrives, grab the emergency kit you've readied for just this eventuality, change into clothes of natural fibers that cover the whole body, put on boots, hop into the car, and tune in for news alerts about the best route to safety.

This is what I've gleaned from residents of California, where the nefarious infernos of 2018 and 2019 displaced hundreds of thousands of people. Those who left quickest had the best chances of survival, for obvious reasons. Less obvious was why some houses burned down and others didn't. Owners of the former weren't well prepared, while some homes didn't burn simply by chance or because the owners had hired private firefighters to battle the flames. To enhance the chances that your house will fall into the still-standing category, landscape it with fire prevention in mind. Remove within one hundred feet of the building anything combustible, such as wooden furniture, dried leaves, and even green vegetation. Install gravel on the outdoor property, water hoses with a long reach, and roofs made of noninflammable materials like tile. Cut off branches within ten feet of the ground to prevent the fire from jumping into trees.

If a fire breaks out, close the windows and doors of the house and shut off gas valves. Move furniture away from windows and remove flammable material like curtains. If possible, stay on the ground level and look out the window, in order to monitor the progress of the fire. Smoke rises so you want to stay low. Fill the bathtub and sinks with water to douse flames. If the fire and smoke make it unsafe to remain in the house any longer, jump into the pool, if you're so lucky to have one. However, falling debris and smoke may ultimately make it unsafe. If fleeing by car, shut windows and air vents. Smoke impairs visibility, so turn on the headlights and keep the doors unlocked for an easy escape. Remain inside if fire approaches the vehicle; this will provide a greater chance of survival. In the unfortunate event that you find yourself without cover, look for bodies of water or open spaces like fields. Lie facedown, preferably on moist soil or mud, in order to breathe cooler air. Don't cover your face with a wet cloth, as the vapor can harm the lungs by transmitting heat. And never, ever run or drive toward flames.

Heat-resistant tents like those used by firefighters can provide some protection for a short period, by creating a pocket of air and reflecting radiant heat. They do not guarantee survival, however, as we saw with the nineteen firemen who died while using them in Arizona a few years back. The shelters fail when in direct contact with flames and should be deployed only in open spaces far away from trees. Don't get a false sense of security by crawling into one.

Earthquakes

We're all waiting for the Big One to hit Southern California, with seismologists predicting a massive jolt sometime in the next thirty years. We're not just worried about the immediate impact, which could topple buildings, destroy highways, and derail trains. Debris or an entire house could bury you. Common complications after a tremor can be equally

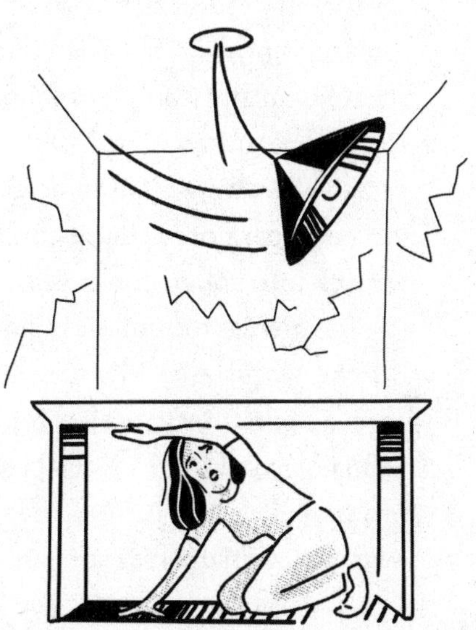

deadly, such as a tsunami, aftershocks, fires, electrocution from exposed and wet wires, and water, sewage, and gas leaks. Your best options are to keep abreast of forecasts by scientists, ready an emergency kit, and know where to seek shelter. Now's the time to anchor heavy furniture to the wall and practice "drop, cover, and hold on."

First, the warning signs. I experienced several of these in Mexico and was always struck by how the animals signaled that quakes were coming. Dogs howled seconds or even minutes before the ground shook. Scientists say that ants and snakes leave their burrows weeks beforehand, which on the bright side saves money on exterminators if your kitchen, like mine, is infested. Eyeing ants is probably not a practical earthquake-tracking mechanism, however. But if Rover paces anxiously, pay heed to his early warning system and get ready to dive under a sturdy table. People have asked me, "What constitutes 'sturdy'?" Jump on it to see if it cracks, and keep a pillow handy to cover your head in case it does. If you can't find a table, then duck by a structural interior wall that hopefully won't crumble. Stay away from windows, ceiling lamps, mirrors, and anything else that might collapse on you. I was always told to head for the nearest doorway, until an engineer noted that it could give way, too. The door could smack into you or the frame crash down.

The advice to remain inside doesn't apply to many parts of the world, like Mexico City, that have lax construction codes or architecture that is poorly engineered to withstand a major shudder. In such places, you run the risk of being entombed in a pancake collapse and are better off fleeing outside to an open space.

Small foreshocks that rattle windows and shelves can herald the onset of something bigger. Pay heed if folks are speculating about UFOs. Earthquake survivors have reported strange lights hovering above the ground. Geophysicists differ on whether this is a true phenomenon related to electric charges released from the earth or something more mundane, like a shaking power line. I'm of the "Be alert to any weird shit" school of thought.

Beware of aftershocks. They can occur hours or days after the first shake. In the unfortunate event that you're trapped under debris, resist the temptation to yell. This may seem counterintuitive, but hollering will deplete your strength and open your airways to dust. Instead, cover your mouth and pull out the spiffy whistle that you always have on your person in case of emergency, or bang on whatever is around you.

Tsunamis

These watery cousins of earthquakes can wreak even more destruction. A giant water surge can measure up to one hundred feet, although even one-tenth of that can cause severe destruction and loss of life. If you don't drown, your car and home may be swept away. Power, roads, and communications may be cut off for days afterward. Red flags include a sharp rise in coastal waters and an ocean roar resembling the sound of a jet engine. Again, follow animals' cue. If they start racing to higher ground inland, so should you. Be on high alert if the sea or ocean suddenly recedes dramatically from the shore. This is not the time to hunt for conch shells newly exposed. Hundreds of fish flapping on wet sand could be the cue to flee to more elevated ground, preferably two miles inland or one hundred feet above sea level. Failing that, climb a tree and hug it tightly, whether or not you're an environmental activist. Praying can't hurt. Provided you survive the first impact, don't go back to the beach just yet. Tsunamis generally come in waves (pun intended), over minutes, hours, or days.

Oregon and parts of California sound the alarm once the seabed cracks open, through sirens, texts, or both. Depending on the location of the underwater quake, the warning means a wave could be hours or minutes away. Now's the time to take note of evacuation routes and time the run, in case you have to make it one day.

Mud- and Landslides

Land- and mudslides can occur anywhere in the United States, triggered by earthquakes or heavy rain on slopes denuded by fire. Rumbling and cracking trees and telephone poles forewarn a slide's advance. The debris and mud can bury towns. You cannot outrun a wall of earth moving at sixty miles an hour; sometimes a slide takes just a minute to rumble down. That's why it's critical to evacuate if given sufficient advance warning. If you happen to have not gotten the advisory, get away from the path of the slide. If stuck inside a building, go to the highest floor or a room that is farthest from the path. Roll into a ball under the furniture.

That being said, foundations of buildings can collapse. So can tunnels and bridges, and roads can wash away, so a car is not necessarily a safe place. When driving, keep in mind that slides can recur, so watch out for falling power lines, trees, telephone poles, debris, and rocks.

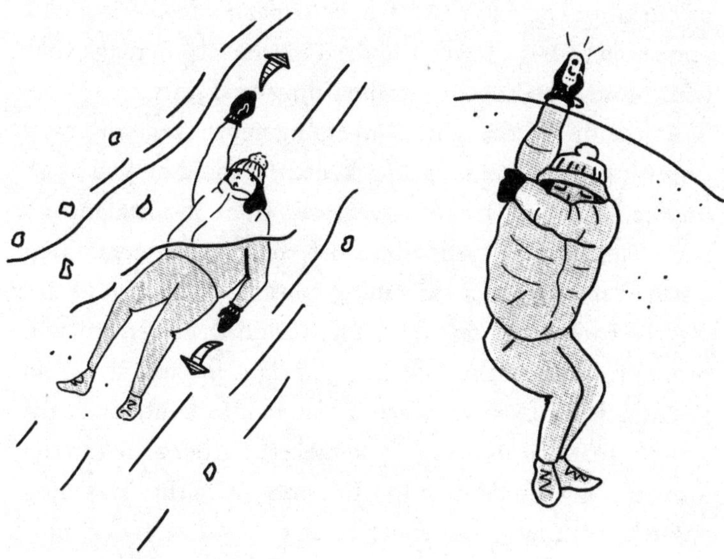

Avalanches

These snowy monsters can move at the speed of a train, with enough force to bury a village. After spending a day avalanche mapping with a Norwegian army team, I vowed never again to snowshoe without a beacon strapped around my shoulder. I learned that even a mere footstep can trigger an avalanche, depending on the slope and layering of snow. The Norwegian experts taught me to check for cracks and previous avalanche activity. Major shifts in weather, like wind, rising temperatures, and recent snowfall, can contribute to instability. Snow barreling down a mountainside makes a frightening *whoomping* sound.

The beacon transceiver can save a life. This radio device emits a pulsed signal that will transmit your location to rescue crews (provided they have a receiver). Firmly attach the beacon onto your person so that you can reach it in case of burial in the snow. Avalanche experts also carry poles and shovels, but I haven't figured out how to manage that while doing sports like snowboarding or skiing.

At the first onslaught of incoming snow, drop all heavy gear (skis, snowshoes, backpack, etc.); it could hit you upon impact. If there's time, move away from the avalanche's path. Failing that, paddle against the current, remaining on the surface with a swimming motion. Think of it as doing the backstroke on snow. This paddling movement will propel you better than plodding upright in deep snow. As the avalanche snow approaches, put your face into one bent arm to create an air pocket, and raise the other arm into the air with a beacon. Stay calm while you create this breathing space by your face. Most people can't stay alive under snow for more than thirty minutes so it's important to conserve energy and oxygen to maximize your chances. Remind yourself that 50 percent of people survive avalanches and think of something pleasant as you wait for someone to notice the beacon. Don't contemplate that they won't.

Volcanoes

As the 1980 eruption of Mount St. Helens showed when it spewed ash on Oregon and Washington, volcanoes are not some mythical thing to prepare for. The United States has nearly 170 active volcanoes, most of them in Alaska. Hawaii is another hot spot, as we saw when Big Island's Kīlauea erupted in 2018. Lava and more than five hundred earthquakes—that's right, five hundred—displaced thousands of residents. Rumbling signals an imminent blowout, as do rising gas and magma and a bulge in the ground. As with wildfires, you absolutely *must* leave the area immediately if warned. Molten rock can race more than sixty miles per hour, and poisonous gas, lava, and rocks can fly for miles. If the lava doesn't kill you, the ash can. Don't ever approach lava flows during an eruption to snap a selfie. Most deaths occur during the pyroclastic flows, a fancy term for fast-moving ash, rock, and toxic gas, or during mudslides afterward. If you haven't been warned, you still have options. There's no point running once the eruption is under way; no one can get ahead of lava. Stay inside until the ash settles, and shut doors, windows, and all sources of ventilation, such as chimneys, furnaces, air conditioners, and fans. Put on long-sleeve tops and trousers and cover your mouth and nose with masks or a dampened cloth. Do the same for the children. Make sure they stay vigilant with those damp cloths.

NUCLEAR AND CHEMICAL HAZARDS

Basically, if you live near a nuclear or chemical plant, or if a rogue state has threatened to send missiles in your direction, take preemptive action today. Ask the local authorities and operating company about contingency and evacuation plans. If they answer, "Um, well . . . ," consider moving to another town. Read up on what a meltdown or spill would look like. Most of us drift along in complacency and figure an explosion won't happen because one hasn't yet. Well, it did in Chernobyl, and thirty years on, children are still being born with defects and disabilities. Hopefully, you won't ever experience a nuclear blowup à la Chernobyl, or get in the way of a nuclear missile, or live near a chemical factory that spews poisons. I really hope that doesn't happen to you. But if it does, race inside immediately and do not go out for at least twenty-four hours—or, better, seventy-two. In particularly lethal cases, you may have to remain indoors for weeks. While that creates tedium, don't budge until authorities give the all-clear. Walls have a remarkable ability to keep out radiation, which grows weaker by the day, so the more time you seek shelter, the better. Stay away from windows and doors through which toxins can leak, and seek out a basement or interior room. Close ventilation sources such as air conditioners. This is not the time to check for roof damage. In the unfortunate event that you're stuck outside, hold a cloth over your mouth and hope for the best. If coming in from outside, remove outer layers of clothing and shoes before entering, so as not to contaminate the space or the other people cowering there. Once inside, thoroughly wash any exposed flesh and hair and change any remaining garments—quickly.

CONCLUSION

There you have it. Assemble the emergency kit, check the weather reports, sign up for alerts, and send the dog to the groomer. It could be a long time until he gets a decent wash. Then power up the generator and wait for the water—or lava flows, or fires, or mud, or dust—to stop.

Now, read on for making the most of your shelter.

Chapter 7

GIMME SHELTER—HUNKERING DOWN WHEN DISASTER STRIKES

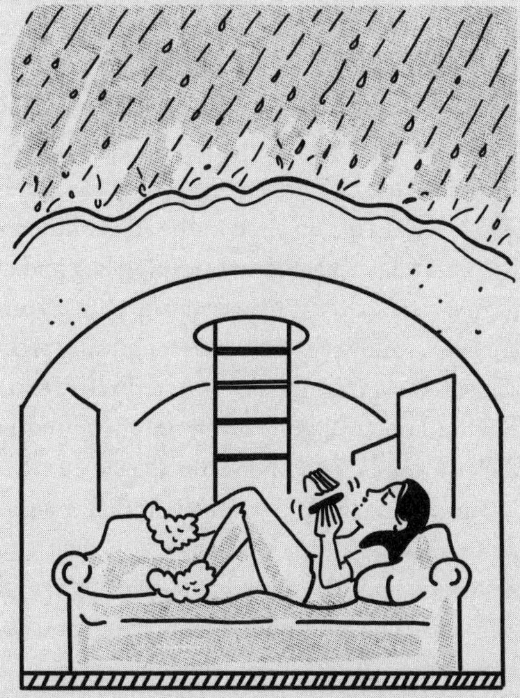

The army bunker on the Colombian mountaintop offered supreme comfort. Unlike some of the other trenches I'd slept in, which were noisy, malarial, or full of scorpions, this one was practically five stars: the Four Seasons, Marquetalia. There, in the soaring heights of the Andes, the government soldiers dug a redoubt into the ground to seek shelter from ambushes by guerrillas. The hiding place, covered with camouflaging leaves, provided just the right dark and quiet for uninterrupted REM—such blissful comfort that I'd never slept sounder, despite being under possible attack. The only noise came from the stalled-truck sound of my own snoring. Earthen bed platforms provided better back support than a Sealy mattress, and a friendly lieutenant stood guard outside, so I wouldn't have to worry about rebels sneaking up and abducting me. He said he'd take care of it. *No problema!*

Except one—a big one. The military encampment had scarce water to wash with, so the body odor of the hundreds of soldiers who preceded me lingered in the trench. The foulness hung in the air and permeated my sleeping bag and clothes. Emerging from the burrow the next morning, I was refreshed and dewy-eyed . . . and reeked like a decomposing pig.

This brings us to a vital lesson: Your experience in a shelter depends on how well you can maintain sound hygiene and morale and ample food and water to ride out the crisis. Hopefully, you will never find yourself on that mountaintop in Marquetalia, or in an air raid shelter, notwithstanding threats of ballistic missiles aimed at Hawaii. What with the changing climate, however, odds are that you, and certainly your children's generation, could face a major natural disaster at some point. An earthquake, tsunami, or hurricane of Katrina proportions could mean being cut off for a week or more. A tornado or biblical flood might confine you to the house, or wherever you happen to be when calamity strikes. If one does, and you are stuck for days or even weeks, try to make the most of an uncomfortable situation. "Prepper" manuals generously share tips on emergency beacons and fuel, but they don't dish on other critical matters, such as keeping armpits fragrant and finding entertainment in a shelter. Whether you are seeking sanctuary in a stadium during a big storm or taking refuge in your own home or on a school floor, you don't have to sacrifice all creature comforts. A bit of preparation will make the ordeal less awful. The key here is to have all the supplies ready ahead of time, so that your basement is cozily equipped when the Apocalypse strikes and you don't have to make runs to Home Depot to purchase a hand-cranked radio as a storm makes landfall. First, be sure you've got the all-purpose emergency kit outlined in chapter 6 ("Do I Stay or Do I Go? Natural Disasters"), including medical supplies, a list of emergency contacts, and spare cash. Then, haul in the heavier gear such as a generator, meals, and entertainment for the home away from home.

THE RIGHT STUFF: FURNISHING YOUR BUNKER

LED FLASHLIGHTS: I like the headlamp variety that shines from your forehead. It frees the hands to do things, such as applying tourniquets and nail polish.

HAND-CRANKED RADIO, SAT PHONE, AND SURGE PROTECTORS: As explained in the previous chapter, these are essential equipment for emergency communications and to maintain a power supply.

GARBAGE BAGS: Self-evident.

CAMPING STOVE: Eating cold survival rations gets tired fast. These nifty, lightweight cookers require no liquids, priming, or wicks. You ignite them with fuel tablets along with solid fuel like hexamine or Sterno. A hot meal will fortify stomachs and spirits, provided you have enough ventilation to avoid being smoked out.

SAD LIGHTS: Some marketers call them "happy lights" or "therapy lights," which sounds more upbeat. The acronym stands for "seasonal affective disorder," which is indeed sad. These strong white lights supposedly lift the mood by replicating natural sunlight. They worked wonders for me during Moscow's interminable winters. The mere four hours of weak daylight per diem sent me, and everyone in my social circle, into a deep funk. Even ordinarily cheerful people, which is not how I would describe myself, had trouble getting out of bed. But the SAD—rather, happy!—lights helped us get moving and maintain a minimal level of activity and sanity. In a similar vein, SAD lights can help combat refuge blues, too—provided you have electricity.

GENERATOR: A must-have for catastrophe furnishings. Stock up on enough fuel for twice the period you expect to hide. How long that might be depends on the type of emergency. A single tornado blows over after ten minutes to an hour, but hurricane stranding can last weeks. As a general rule, prepare for two weeks. This will allow you to plug in the SAD-cum-happy light and recharge cell phones and laptops so you can stay abreast of *Seinfeld* reruns during bomb raids.

SCENTED CANDLES: They have a relaxing effect when one contemplates the catastrophe outside. They'll also provide illumination, and obscure disgusting odors. Just make sure they don't cause a fire, as there's nowhere else to run.

FOND REMINDERS: Bring photos of loved ones who aren't with you, especially pets who adore you unconditionally. People crammed in a shelter quickly get on each other's nerves, and the photos will remind you of happier times.

DISTRACTION BLOCKERS: Prime the environs with earplugs to block out the complaints around you. There will be many, I assure you.

GROSS CORNER: Designate a corner of the space for the dirty stuff—trash, toilet, cat litter, etc. It should be far from the sleeping quarters.

BEDDING: Mattresses can get mildewy in damp, airless spaces, so better to use sleeping bags with liners atop air or foam mattresses.

FAN: If you have a reliable power source, consider fans to circulate the air. This will make for a fresher environment, especially when you're not bathing as often as you normally do.

BUNKER HYGIENE

Even a few hours in a confined space can make a woman (or man) feel, and smell, like a fetid wolverine. Odor molecules ferment, and being cooped up with other noxious bodies stinks, in every sense of the word. Do not despair. One can achieve glamour, or at least minimal sanitary standards, in such circumstances, as I learned from the pros.

These would be Angolans, some of the most stylish, and innovative, people I met during decades of covering combat. Thirty-five years of wartime deprivations taught them how to remain coiffed and fragrant without functional plumbing. I had the opportunity to learn from these wise masters after UNITA insurgents bombed the water supply (yet again) when I was stationed in the country in 1992. Alongside millions of Angolan citizens, I went weeks without running water. At first, I used baby wipes to cleanse, but they left a stale stickiness on my skin, and my supply eventually ran out. In contrast, my Angolan friends exuded aromatic freshness.

I finally got up the nerve to ask one particularly radiant woman her secret. Her skin glowed like moonshine, and her hair caught the sun's glint. How in heaven's name did she manage to stay so unsoiled?

"Booze," she shared conspiratorially. Vodka served as an astringent for greasy pores and scalps. She followed this up with a beer rinse that made the hair glisten. If any libations were left over, she took swigs to calm her nerves during the frequent cross fire in the street outside her bathroom. That kept her brow unfurrowed during stressful moments. "You won't be disappointed," she assured me, fishing a can of lager from her handbag. "Take it everywhere in case you get stuck during a raid."

She was right. I tried this technique in various bath-challenged situations, including just the other week, when the city shut off the water on my street in Manhattan. I can testify to alcohol's power. My hair follicles never looked healthier, and the acne from not showering dried up. My skin had a shine derived not from sweat but deep-cleaned pores. Over time, as I faced water-challenged situations, I experimented with alternative alcoholic beverages. In place of vodka, one can substitute gin, tequila, whisky, brandy, grappa—you get the idea. Any hard liquor will do, although, personally, I favor clear liquids because they remind me of water.

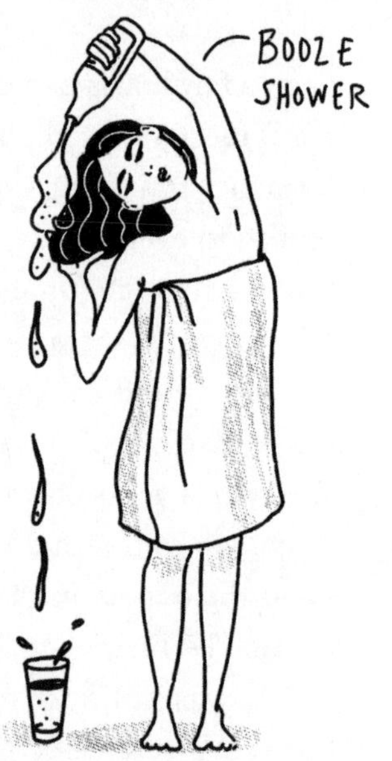

Load up on dental floss. It takes up less room than toothpaste and doesn't require water to clean the teeth. I learned this tip from a South African mercenary, who pointed out that the minty smell of toothpaste can also give away your position if you're hiding in the bush. Even if you're hiding from a tornado in a town, forfeit the Colgate just in case.

Use sanitary pads when menstruating. Don't waste tampons; they're handy for plugging bullet holes. Furthermore, not washing properly encourages the growth of all sorts of funky bacteria that you don't want to push farther inside with a roll of cotton with a string attached. Pads have no age limit; you don't have to have your period to enjoy the benefits of panty liners. They substitute for fresh underwear when the washing machine doesn't work, or exist.

Unless the shelter has access to a bountiful well, water will likely be in short supply. Before you huddle in the cellar or attic, or anywhere, practice bathing from a bucket. I learned the hard way that this refined art requires dress rehearsals in order not to spill precious drops. The way it works is this: you wash with only three cups of water a day—a cup for the sensitive bits, one for armpits, and a spare for the face and hands. You can stretch it to two more for the head, one to soap up and one to rinse—*but only if you don't have alcoholic beverages handy for shampoo.* The trick is to use the bucket sparingly and not hog all the water, so everyone else can wash as well. Such generosity will endear you to your bunker mates, and the environs will be fresher if everyone gets a chance to douse.

Toileting

Al fresco urination poses myriad challenges in myriad situations, for myriad people. While out with NATO troops in the glacial Arctic, I learned that the penis can be frostbitten when pulled out in minus-fifty-five degrees. (Not from personal experience, mind you. I have never had a phallic appendage. This is what male soldiers have told me.) That's why Everest climbers keep "pee bottles" in their tents. These nifty apparatuses can be fashioned from regular water bottles or from jars with an opening big enough to accommodate the stream. Place the container in the correct spot and do the business. Ready-made products like the Freshette work well for women. But beware! Like bucket bathing, bottle pissing requires tryouts so you don't urinate all over your clothes. Some people prefer to stand, some kneel, and others stretch out on their sides. All these positions require practice to ensure the pee doesn't trickle down the legs. Figure out what works best for your knees. Once perfected, this handy skill can be summoned when you don't feel like schlepping to the bathroom in the middle of the night. Keep one by the bed! Just be careful not to mistake it for your cup of water. (Quick note of comfort, though: If you do sip pee, you won't die, and doctors say it's a good way to stay hydrated if you run out of Poland Spring. Fortunately, I've never had to try this, but hey, you've gotta do what you've gotta do.)

Outdoor elimination makes little sense in many other situations. During a nuclear strike, eyes can be blinded if turned toward a fireball, and radiation will burn the skin on exposed butts. If facing a more conventional land attack, as I was on that Colombian mountain, someone could sneak up and shoot you in the privates—with the added indignity of your pants pulled down to your knees. Throughout tsunamis, you could be swept out to sea. As for earthquakes, a traffic light or a building could collapse on you during aftershocks.

Finally, aside from making you vulnerable to ambushes, outdoor latrines attract nasty vermin. When I was in a Sudan People's Liberation Army rebel camp in South Sudan, we had to do our business over a hole in the ground swarming with scorpions. I quickly learned to be quick and efficient and always to wear boots. The same goes for rattlesnakes, other snakes, poisonous spiders, poison ivy, and anything else that creeps you out. Also, check that the privy is constructed soundly. I still shudder over a nightmarish scenario during the civil war in Zaire in 1996, when a flimsy outhouse collapsed around a colleague relieving her bladder. She fell neck-deep into the filthy privy and was sick for months afterward. Kids have drowned in rickety outhouses in South Africa.

To avoid such calamities, install a potty pail indoors. This glorified chamber pot can be fashioned from a toilet bowl or a five-gallon container lined with two sturdy garbage bags. Put cat litter or sawdust at the bottom of the bags to offset the stench, and secure them tightly at the end of the day. Keep this unsanitary device far from sleeping and eating areas. If it's safe to pop outside the shelter occasionally, hurl the bags far from the entrance, but not so forcefully that they burst. And remember what Mom said: Always wash your hands, preferably with antiseptic wipes, after toilet use and before eating.

DRESS FOR SUCCESS

For lack of a minibar, wrap hair with a turban or scarf, preferably of cotton, which absorbs sweat better than synthetics. Head covers have the added benefit of diverting lice.

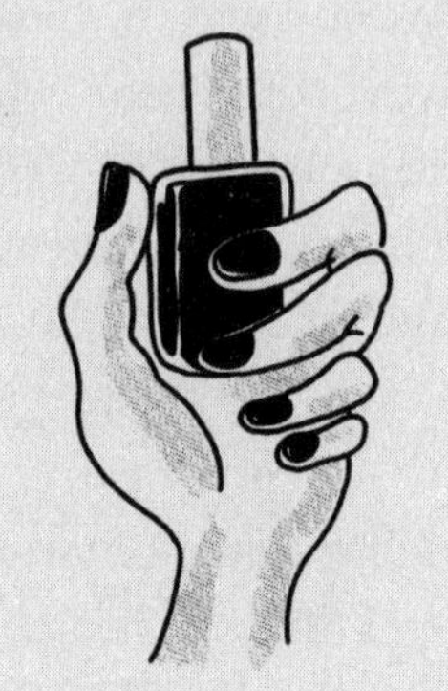

Until the 1950s, average Americans washed their hair only once a week. That changed when the geniuses on Madison Avenue realized they could sell more shampoo if people used it daily. Most scalps can last a month without developing a serious skin disease.

In a waterless emergency, I paint my nails a dark color in order to obscure filth. I avoid reds after once mistaking my red nail polish for blood when I groggily woke up. I'm partial to dark blues like China Glaze's "Up All Night"—which is what I am during a crisis. The navy sheen looks less funereal than black. And lest you think I'm being petty or tongue-in-cheek, consider this: During the Blitz, the British government encouraged civilians to keep up their physical appearances in order to maintain morale. I've found that a manicure is an excellent way to distract oneself from the threat of losing one's house to a storm or whatever, although anxiety can cause hands to shake, thus risking getting polish on the fingers.

I prefer to wear basic black clothes in extreme situations, with the exceptions of the riots and heat I mentioned earlier. I take my cue from Parisian war correspondents, who always choose that color whether or not they're at the frontlines. There's an added practical point to consider besides feeling chic. Aside from making a fashion statement, black hides grime—your wardrobe will accumulate dirt no matter how many vodka body rinses you perform. This is how I got by—and, heck, I wanted to make sure I still looked thin while not exercising and after gorging on survival biscuits all day out of boredom.

Continuing on the French riff, I emulate unwashed noblewomen from the Middle Ages and drench myself in perfume. I spray it everywhere to mask foul odors. *Everywhere*. Vodka mist works well for this, too. Mix one part vodka with two parts water in a spray bottle, add your favorite essential oil, and spritz away! This solution can also deodorize stinky mattresses and pillows that get moldy in the shelter.

BUNKER ETIQUETTE AND FUN (OR NOT)

Fun—there ain't much of it in a crisis. Camaraderie in an airless, confined space becomes hard to maintain as time drags on. Tempers grow as ripe as bodies stuck side by side, even in a substantial basement. Pleasantries quickly disappear, especially when someone takes a dump in the wash bucket (see "Bunker Hygiene"). Critical levels of stress build up, as the person sitting next to you morphs into an enemy who ate all the remaining tuna fish.

Don't let the cramped experience interfere with creative juices. Now's a good opportunity to write that novel you always talked about. You'll find lots of solitude when everyone refuses to speak to one another. However, this is not the time to take up the guitar. No one wants to hear you practice chords, or sing tunelessly. Leave all instruments at home, especially the winds (e.g., the tuba), which require extra oxygen.

Fortify yourself with yoga and meditation, or any other

exercise that can be practiced quietly with eyes closed, so you don't have to look at the annoying people sharing the small space.

Board games and playing cards help pass the time. Dominoes take up little space, as do travel chess sets. However, I don't recommend Monopoly. The emphasis on real estate will serve as a bitter reminder of the tight space, and "Go to Jail" hits too close to home. Apropos, prisoners in Russia sometimes organize talks to make productive use of the time. Cellmates give lectures on their areas of expertise. Topics could include languages, political theory, and interior design.

BUNKER PETS

As we all know, people have difficulty parting with their dogs and cats during natural disasters. Don't be surprised if a Labrador pops up in a shelter during a crisis, and pack Benadryl if you suffer from dog allergies. Getting it to poop in the potty pail poses problems, as you can well imagine. Pets require a designated place to do their business, far from the sleeping zone. If you're worried about carbon monoxide poisoning from lack of ventilation, take a caged canary or finch along. Coal miners used to use the birds

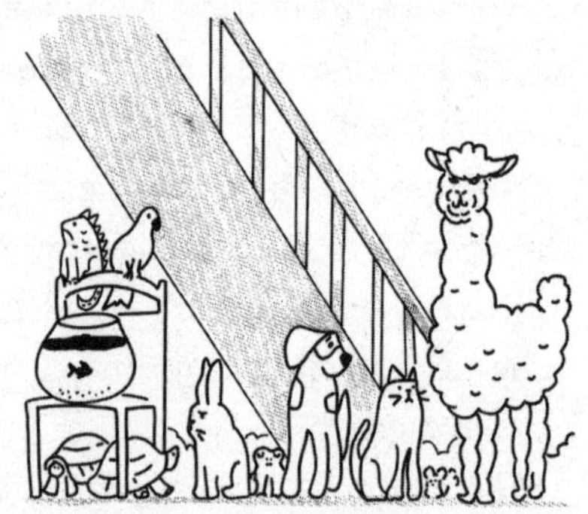

for early detection of noxious gases, as they are more sensitive to fumes than humans. If the canary grows weak or dies, consider evacuating the shelter.

BUNKER DINING

As a general rule during any calamity, mobilize enough food and water for at least two weeks. (Being a glass-half-empty kind of person, I would routinely stockpile double or triple that amount.) It's always wise to err on the side of extreme panic.

Water—you can go without bathing and sunlight, but not hydrating. Everyone needs to drink water in order to live. Budget one gallon per person per day. That accounts for their cooking, washing, and drinking needs. Of course, fourteen gallons per person for a fortnight, the average amount of time to prepare for, is a lot of water that has to be stored somewhere. Whenever we anticipated water shortages, we filled up the bathtub. Generally, bathtubs in hotels where I was holed up were on the smaller side, meaning they could hold about thirty-five gallons (or slightly over two weeks' worth of water for one person). Bigger ones in American homes can handle eighty gallons. Once the tub was filled, we would scoop water to flush the toilet (if it still worked) and wash. Don't drink bathwater—it probably has residue from cleaning fluids and soap that could cause indigestion, or worse. Water filters might work in a pinch, but I much prefer to stockpile giant canisters and pallets of bottled water for drinking purposes. Any leftovers can be sold on eBay or used to wash the car.

As for food, when heading to the front, I routinely packed MREs. For those unfamiliar with military vernacular, these are Meals, Ready-to-Eat, otherwise known as "Meals Rarely Edible." They taste and look like something the cat threw up. War crimes should be declared against these ghastly offerings of mush. Such dining abominations, however, come in vacuum-sealed packages and afford all the nutrition needed to survive, which is why soldiers carry them on combat missions when far from mess halls. I gnawed on MREs when besieged in a starving town, where land mines planted by the enemy prevented trucks from bringing in food supplies. I took MREs to Rwanda after the genocide, to avoid paying exorbitant restaurant bills. I've eaten them while camping. Sadly, MREs sold through civilian camping stores and websites are as unappetizing as the military varieties. There's one advantage, however. Because of the appalling lack of flavor, you may want to eat only once a day, which will cut down enormously on food storage (and cost) and help you knock off a few pounds!

Each package generally consists of a main dish, a side, and a "dessert," with some sort of drink mixture. MREs can be warmed with a flameless ration heater that is water activated, or not. Whatever the serving temperature, they're awful, but some of the meals taste better than others (although not by much). My confidential military sources report that the Chili Mac and Cheese and the Maple Sausage are the most palatable, but that one should avoid the Omelet, otherwise known as the "Vomelet." The American fighting man has been known to throw punches on the frontlines as he scrambles for the best offerings. I advise ordering European options online, as the Old World offers finer cuisine on the battlefront, as one would expect from Continental chefs. It's the closest you'll get to bistro dining. Portuguese military rations offer proper tuna packed in olive oil, and the Italians' pasta actually resembles pasta. But the best MREs I ever swallowed were the Norwegian army's. The lamb curry and Thai fish were to die for—so to speak.

In addition to their distinct lack of appeal, MREs stop up the digestive system. But don't try to counteract that by eating prunes! Constipation is actually the shelterer's best friend, because there's no flow if you can't go. Thus, the toilet bucket fills up slowly. One can always sort out regularity upon resurfacing into polite society.

If you're stashing ordinary food, opt for canned and dry stuff that doesn't require refrigeration. And don't believe what you read on food labels. Many items remain edible well past the expiry date. If vacuum-packed, white rice can last up to twenty-five years (brown rice, far less, as it holds in more moisture). Nonfat powdered milk and most grains are good for a decade. Unopened boxed Cheerios can last up to eight months after the sell-by; sealed containers of processed peanut butter, a bit longer. (The natural kind will go rancid quicker.) Canned tuna and Spam are safe for five years; some people say they can keep for even thirty, but I haven't tested that. Pasta stored correctly remains edible for more than twenty. Rumor has it that salt and sugar can last forever with the right ventilation to prevent mold. (I've heard Twinkies can, too, but don't rush to stockpile them until you've confirmed this with a scientist.)

Cats and dogs in a bunker have it hard, unless they want to eat human meals, which could have dire effects on the litter box. Canned pet food is fatty and oily, which makes it go bad quickly. Oxygen absorbers for some reason don't work with dry pet food, which develops mold and ruins everything else in the container. If any food, pet or human, smells bad when you open it, throw it away. Same with cans that are punctured or swollen, the telltale signs of botulism.

By all means, avoid the example of the former owner of my house in Manhattan, a preacher who had a sound understanding of theology but not food science. The minister expected the Apocalypse and amassed twenty outsize buckets of beans, rice, and assorted grains in the basement for when Judgment Day arrived. In theory, cool and dark places are optimal for food's longevity; however, the minister failed to squirrel these items away properly. Light, mice, and moisture ruined the emergency supplies. Bugs squiggled inside, and everything grew moldy and stale. The End of Days, for the food at least, arrived in 2000, when my husband and I tossed everything into the Hudson River.

With this in mind, make sure your survival food is dry and the containers airtight against oxygen and heat. Had our preacher used Mylar bags with oxygen absorbers, which are packets of iron powder that encourage nitrogen, the canned goodies would still be ready for use come Doomsday. A room temperature of fifty degrees Fahrenheit is ideal. Don't, as the minister did, store it by the boiler.

DIG IT (SHELTERS)

Few of us have personal silos built to withstand a nuclear strike. My second cousin Barbie certainly doesn't where she lives in Hawaii. She emailed me in a panic after the false report of an inbound ballistic missile from North Korea last January. The text from authorities helpfully advised citizens to "SEEK IMMEDIATE SHELTER."

"But where?" a rattled Barbie asked.

My personal experience did not extend to strikes by Kim Jong-un, so I canvassed disaster experts for tips. Their suggestion? Barbie should prime a shelter in her basement. That meant filling up all the water bottles, grabbing Fido, and locking the doors upstairs to keep out any possible looters.

There was one problem: Hawaiians generally don't have cellars because homes there are generally built on lava rock, and it would cost a fortune to blast it with explosives. Houses not constructed on this hard "blue" rock lie on filled-in marshland, which is equally unfeasible for basement construction due to instability and the tendency to attract centipedes.

Not having a basement creates a predicament, of course. One has at most fifteen minutes to take cover in a nuclear event, and unfortunately most American cities long ago deactivated the nuclear shelters that were set up during the Cold War. That being the case, I researched alternatives for Second Cousin Barbie. The findings:

Start digging, whatever the cost—like, the day you move in.

Move to a house with a basement.

Move to an upper-floor apartment in a high building where you can take shelter in the center, away from windows.

Pressure elected officials to designate safe hiding places next to the house.

Time how long it takes to get to a tunnel or a hotel with a parking garage.

Provided you can find shelter from radiation, hopefully you had the foresight to bring duct tape to seal windows, doors, and vents. Tune into emergency alerts on your hand-cranked radio—if things outside are really bad, authorities may warn you to stay put for a very long time. Then settle in and hope someone else eats the Omelet MRE.

IT'S ALL OKAY

Let's say the dreaded Apocalypse doesn't occur. Cold water fills the tub, and the larder bulges with five months' worth of boxed ziti. This happened to us in Moscow, when we prepared for nuclear meltdown during the Y2K fears at the end of the last millennium. As mentioned earlier, nothing happened. At first, I felt foolish, but you know what? Better safe than sorry, and I didn't have to shop for groceries for a long time. If this happens to you, make lots of pasta salad, do laundry, and enjoy your indoor plumbing.

Chapter 8

DRINKING

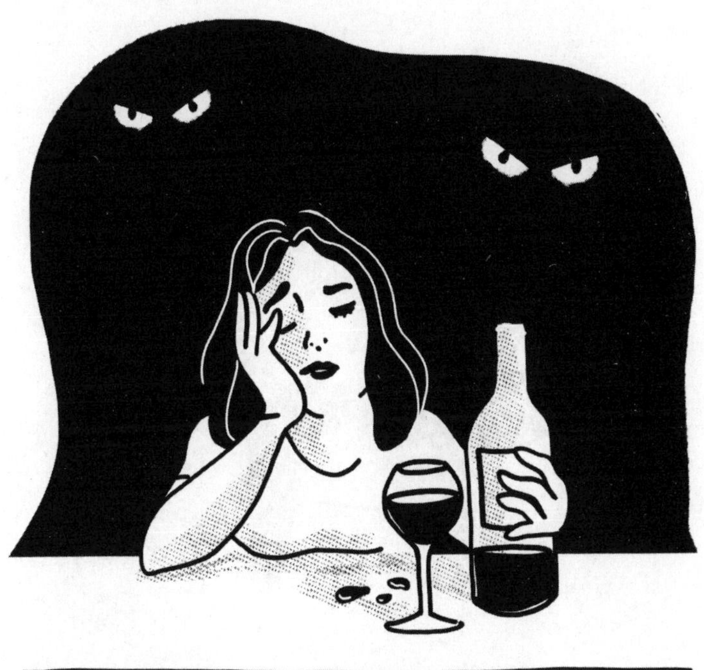

Problematic.

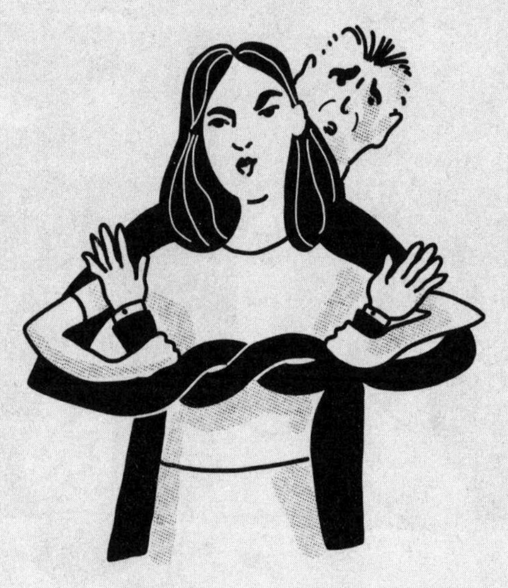

Chapter 9

#METOO AND RAPE

Whenever I'm on assignment, rape looms among my biggest fears, and not rape by some random stranger. I most fear attacks by someone I encounter through work: translators, fixers, drivers, bosses, policemen, soldiers, cameramen, photographers, subordinates, peers, and interview subjects on whom I depend professionally. Statistics bear out that I have reason to be concerned, as should all women. A woman in America is raped approximately every six minutes, and one in five will be sexually assaulted at some point. The number is higher in many countries. Most attackers are someone they know. Realistically, you are more likely to encounter a coworker knocking on your hotel room door or that creepy dude who decides you're his best friend with benefits. Still, we often have trouble accepting that rape and harassment come from people we know, that our worst nightmare is not some unfamiliar person standing next to us in the elevator, but rather someone we had a date with two nights ago.

Then there are the less dangerous but equally disturbing advances. Women, and sometimes men, face obnoxious and demeaning comments from all manner of acquaintances, particularly those in positions of power. We often put up with it because we are conditioned not to confront them or we fear retribution. Ideally, we want to deescalate in the calmest way possible, to protect not only our physical selves but also our future interactions. As the Me Too movement's revelations have shown, harassment cuts across all professions, from big-name movie stars to waitresses to female physicians. I'd like to think that the situation has improved since my days as a young reporter in London, when I'd go to the pub and overhear coworkers speaking in vivid anatomical detail about women they wanted to bonk. Regrettably, even now I still hear the same crude banter when such people think female colleagues aren't listening.

In addition to debasing and lecherous comments, I've faced my share of gropes and hand grazes. One news editor asked about my sexual partners during the annual review of my professional performance. While discussing options for promotion and the impact of my stories, he boomed, "Hey, Matloff. What's the bed situation?" When I was starting out my career, and in my twenties, another male supervisor followed me into a restaurant ladies' room during a working lunch. A bathroom! I didn't consider sex with him appealing in *any location*. When I rebuffed his advances, he grew surly, and once back at the office, he launched a relentless campaign to undermine my work. Fortunately, I got transferred to another country before he could sabotage my career, but the thought that he could have inflicted lasting damage was sobering, indeed.

What really shook me, though, and taught me critical lessons about the need for preparation for all levels of aggravation, from remarks to assault, was the time I flew to a diamond-smuggling area in western Africa with a female colleague. We wanted to look into human rights abuses by the rogue general who controlled the area. No one had yet verified rumors that he forced the locals into slave labor to pan for stones that eventually became engagement rings on American fingers. The general had a brutish reputation, as did the goons who served on the local police force. My friend and I thought we were clever to talk our way onto the light aircraft of a gem trafficker and then naïvely figured we could handle any bad situation that might transpire once we deplaned into thug territory. I might add that this was in the early 1990s, before the advent of cell phones and the internet. And because the sat phone weighed too much to lug aboard, we had no way to send SOS messages in case something went wrong.

Which it did.

Upon landing on the dirt patch that approximated a landing strip, the pilot hurriedly picked up his precious package of contraband and flew off with the ominous words "I wouldn't linger if I were you." As the plane shrank to a speck in the sky, two policemen approached, aiming their rusty AK-47 rifles. They leered drunkenly. They cackled. They debated enthusiastically who was going to march which of us into the shack one hundred yards away. I froze. My life didn't exactly fly by with scenes from the past; instead, I imagined the final frame, where my limp, mutilated corpse spurted blood like in a vampire movie. While I hyperventilated over this picture of a hideous end, my level-headed colleague stalled the inebriated evildoers with made-up logic. Harming us would cause a diplomatic incident, she coolly informed them. (Not true.) The general himself was waiting for us. (Also not true.)

We were *terribly important* people. (Definitely not true.) They should get the defense minister on the phone to confirm that fact. She failed to mention that we were bit players whom nobody but our parents cared about, but in such circumstances, a bit of exaggeration's okay, and could even be a lifesaver. Being soused, the guardians of the peace required extra time to process the information. Granted, it was a lot to take in even for a sober individual, and these two were having difficulty simply standing. While they debated the chances of being caught and losing their jobs, and whether it was better just to throw us into the river, a deus ex machina appeared, just like in a Hollywood movie: A priest roared up out of nowhere in a beat-up vehicle and ordered the police to step back. Being God-fearing Catholics, they obeyed, and we jumped into the Father's vehicle. I considered converting.

The incident terrified me. I was damned lucky. Divine intervention is not a safety precaution, so learning to set firm boundaries was at the top of my list when I later began teaching younger generations better safety than I had practiced. So many lessons emerged from this unpleasant incident that I carried them forward into more mundane situations. Today, I would try to avoid an isolated area, or even a city street, without first establishing an escape route or a communications setup. While there's little defense against two thugs with rifles, my pal had wisely deescalated, or at least slowed down, the situation by negotiating with them until help arrived. With that in mind, I began to research the best way to teach women to set strong psychological, verbal, and physical barriers.

Granted, the episode I've just described was extreme, but we all have fears of menacing circumstances occurring, such as being assaulted by a guy you've met at a party, or having your taxi driver stop the car and force himself on you. But I share this story because it was my reckoning with myself, and it forced me to think about what I could do in similar situations. I made some bad choices, and I didn't think things through. It was a real wake-up call.

Whether you're on assignment in Africa or on a date gone wrong, the fear is the same. Assault is not the fault of the victim, but knowing ways to protect yourself is important in order to stay safe. Unfortunately, the onus is often on us women to take action. Reactions to threats of rape and harassment and how one deals with the aftermath are varied, but they all require a mind-set that you're not helpless. There are strategies you can follow. Dodging situations likely to put you in a dangerous or uncomfortable position in the first place is important. Failing that, the key is to try to shift the balance of power. The self-defense trainer I work with suggests flexing control in everyday low-stakes interactions, in order to get used to being more assertive. So many women feel uncomfortable pushing their own agendas, so it requires a bit of practice. Here are some scenarios to start with.

HARASSMENT

Make Clear It's Not Cool

A jerk leans in close. He puts his arm on your shoulder, with the hand dangling ominously close to your bosom. It's one of those "Am I misreading his intentions?" moments. You probably aren't, and even if he's simply an elderly man who feels an Old World need to physically express warmth, that touch makes you uneasy—period. Trust your gut. If you feel uncomfortable, there's probably a reason, and you have a right to convey that. Depending on the scenario, several approaches exist to dodge the paw:

- Move back a pace. Once, I walked backward the entire length of a ballroom to maintain an appropriate distance from a grabby French politician. He kept trying to paw my arm. I managed to keep a foot ahead.
- Tell him you have personal space issues, or that you have the flu and he shouldn't get too near. Invent a prickly condition on the arm/shoulder/back/etc. that should not be touched. ("Hey! I have poison ivy/ burns/eczema/ arthritis/a broken collarbone.")
    - If *that* fails, physically remove the annoying hand. Take his hand off your body and place it on *his*. The guy will likely be so startled that he won't try it again.
- Make a joke (even though it's not funny). Examples:
    - "Hey, you could be arrested for that."
    - "My husband/boyfriend/partner/employer won't like this."
    - "I'd be fired if I pulled that on you."

All these are intended to set boundaries without escalating an uncomfortable situation into a confrontation. By keeping things light, you're signaling your displeasure in a face-saving way. That said, you could look him straight in the eye and in a clear, calm voice say, "Please stop," and then hold that eye contact until he looks away. Repeat "stop" if he doesn't get the message at first. That often does the trick.

Dealing with Catcalls

I don't get these much anymore since I hit pension age, one of the perks of growing older, but I certainly suffered my share of irritating pickup lines during the bloom of youth. Most women have. A 2014 study by Cornell University of more than sixteen thousand women around the world found that 84 percent had experienced street harassment before the age of seventeen. In the United States, 72 percent of women said they took alternative transportation due to harassment. (See Resources.)

Catcalls are the most common form of harassment and are hard to deal with because they're so haphazard. Strangers know they can get away with them. I suggest striding past with confidence and ignoring them, especially if on a dark or empty street. That way you deny the finks what they most want, a reaction. Snapping back often leads to even worse comments, so just walk on by. Some women wear earphones without switching them on, in order to give the impression that they can't hear. If harassed in front of a store, go in and loudly inform the shopkeeper in earshot of other customers that the unwanted attention is bad for business. Someone might go out and tell the harasser to scram.

Avert Annoying Come-ons

One of the old chestnuts I used to hear was "You have beautiful eyes." While that's not overtly sexual, it often signals that further observations, about parts of the body lower down, in the T and A department, will follow. Unlike with catcalls, I generally find that ignoring such remarks doesn't work. For that reason, I favor unexpected responses that throw the dynamic off-kilter, such as "The pink eye infection brings out the blue." Then immediately introduce another topic. It's a nonconfrontational way to convey that you don't appreciate such comments. If he persists, make clear that you want him to stop.

Deflect with Alternatives

We all know that guy. The one who just cannot hear "no" no matter how many ways you say it. He insists on taking you out for a drink or a meal. This happens to me frequently on business trips—still. One senior military source in Burundi tried to persuade me to go out for dinner after the curfew that had been imposed by his army. I pointed out that there were orders to shoot anyone outside after dark. He pointed out that his men enforced the curfew, and he could order the restaurant to stay open and soldiers not to shoot us en route. Obviously, I didn't want to go out alone with a senior military man whose army committed atrocities, even before curfew. A more innocuous situation I often encountered: the guy says he wants to show you the town or take you out, and he gives off a too-intimate vibe. Or you just don't think it's a good idea to go to bars with a business contact.

Politely decline with an excuse about work: "I need to edit at least eight hundred pages by tomorrow morning." This reminds the person that you're in town for business. Then quickly follow up with a neutral suggestion, like meeting for a meal or coffee in the lobby restaurant, where you'd be surrounded by dozens of other customers. That way you don't get trapped in a vehicle with him, somewhere far from your lodging. Don't order alcohol for yourself, as that can muddy your responses and send an unintended message that this is a social meeting, which it isn't. If you have an expense account, insist on picking up the tab. Paying hits home that you're calling the shots—and not doing them. When you're done with your nonalcoholic Diet Coke, walk him to the front entrance to ensure he doesn't try to follow you up to your room.

Set Boundaries with Work Contacts

Like many women in other fields, I face a huge dilemma. I rely on business contacts to share information. Alienating overly flirtatious sources could hurt my ability to report stories. At the same time, I want to keep everything on a professional plane. As advised in an earlier chapter, drink alcohol in moderation only, and try to avoid seeing the person alone in a hotel room or office. Instead, make appointments for a public place like a Starbucks. Bring along a colleague. If the vibe gets too weird for comfort, inform your supervisor, both verbally and in writing, that the source is acting improperly. Once, I invited my boss to a meeting with a press flak of the Polisario Front, the Sahrawi liberation movement in Morocco, who wanted to discuss my personal life instead of the group's political strategy. As I wasn't getting much out of the meetings besides feeling annoyed, I didn't have much to lose, and I felt a measure of control by handing him over to someone else.

SPOTLIGHT ON PAPER TRAILS

Harassers think they can get away with bad behavior for lack of witnesses. Not so fast, Buster. There's email. Send him a "Dear John" message along the lines of:

Dear [insert harasser's name]:

I value our professional relationship and our work collaboration. However, I felt uncomfortable last night in the [office/bar/restaurant/office party] at [specific time and place] when you [tried to kiss me/touched my butt/back/breast/thigh/waist/asked me to sleep with you/asked about my boyfriend/stuck your hand in my shirt/up my skirt/etc.].

I would hate for this incident to jeopardize the productivity of our work environment. I trust it will not happen again, so that we can regain our professional footing. I also trust that there will be no repercussions because I called this to your attention.

Sincerely,
[Your full name]

Blind-copy yourself, using your personal email address (to have a copy accessible in case of any retaliatory measures) and hit Send. The harasser ought to realize that the message can be copied to everyone in the office.

If a coworker or supervisor is doing the harassing, report the incident to Human Resources, with the full understanding that HR is generally more interested in protecting the organization than an employee who got felt up at the water cooler. As insurance against retaliatory action, communicate your complaint to a trusted colleague before setting up a meeting, and then bring said confidante along. You both will take notes. You will also hand over to HR a meticulous record of offensive occurrences, with names, dates, times, and screenshots of the offending emails, photos, and texts. Mine your inner journalist. Come armed with facts, facts, facts. Prepare the dossier even if the company lacks an HR department. Employees of companies that hire at least fifteen people have protections from harassment and discrimination under Title VII, a federal law. If you work for a smaller firm, report the incidents to supervisors and consider hiring a lawyer, or casually mention that you're seeking legal counsel.

Or you could go to the police and ask to wear a wire like Ambra Battilana Gutierrez, one of Harvey Weinstein's alleged victims. After reporting a groping incident in 2015 to the police, she consented with law enforcement to confront Weinstein while secretly recording him. Voila! Weinstein admitted to touching her inappropriately, giving her the evidence needed to lodge charges against him.

Enlist Allies

My workshops include mixed-gender training, and I'm always struck by the horrified looks on the men's faces when the women swap "he did that" stories. Men often don't realize what we endure or know how we'd like them to intervene. For a long time, I tried to hide my vulnerability with quips and bravado in order to fit in with macho male coworkers. But that doesn't help others understand women's problems. Instead, share your stories, and be direct with potential male allies about how you'd want them to intervene in a given situation, be it telling the offender that his behavior is inappropriate or creating a physical barrier between you and a catcaller. Do you want the men with you to act like protectors? To refrain from engaging in bro talk? Tell them. As for identifying good allies, generally, the guys who seem evolved when it comes to gender roles will be the ones you'll instinctively trust or feel comfortable with in social situations. Such dudes are more likely to gain your sympathy and want to help.

While you're rustling up good guys to serve as allies, spread the word about offenders among female colleagues. Chances are you're not the only woman being harassed. Female journalists have informal lists of offenders, and we warn one another to stay away or maintain a cautious distance. Canvass others to ascertain whether a given person is a serial harasser, and get out the word for others to be on the alert around him. "Me Too" means just that.

RAPE

Safety in Numbers and Drinking

Two conditions are the best friends of assault: isolation and binge drinking. While assault is never the victim's fault, unfortunately, women must be aware of what can happen when we leave ourselves vulnerable, and we must learn what strategies work best to protect us.

Whenever possible, avoid being alone with a man you don't trust or know well. This is stupendously hard for journalists to do, as we're often working on our own. Still, we are less likely to be attacked with witnesses present. I have some hard-and-fast rules for myself: I steer clear of holding meetings in hotel rooms, and whenever possible I avoid going to an unfamiliar man's house for interviews, or going on drives in his car, particularly in strange and remote places where I can't easily hop out and call for help. Public places like coffee shops are preferable venues to meet. As an extra precaution, I ask someone to call me during the course of the get-together—sometimes several times, if I'm feeling really uneasy. I pick up the phone with the words, "I'm meeting with Mr. Smith at X location. I'll call you in an hour, as soon as I'm done." That sends the message to the man that someone knows you're there and expects to hear from you at a set time. If you continue to feel uncomfortable, tell the man this and make an exit. Trust your instincts.

As for drinking, don't try to keep up with the guys if you're at dinner or a party. Women metabolize alcohol differently from men. Whatever we imbibe takes longer for our bodies to break down than a man's, and it causes higher blood-alcohol levels. In other words, we get drunk quicker and stay drunk longer. According to the Centers for Disease Control and Prevention, research suggests that heavy drinking is a risk factor especially at college, where one in twenty women is assaulted. The CDC cites studies showing that more than 70 percent of women who report being raped were under the influence at the time. Perps count on the dulling effects of substances to make women more vulnerable to their attacks, so aside from knowing your limits, don't leave your drink unattended at a bar or party, to guard against someone slipping in a rape drug that incapacitates. If you forget and step away from your drink, order a new one when you return.

Self-Defense

Weapons can be as dangerous as they might be protective. After all, what you bring to a fight can and very likely will be used against you. The pro: You have a knife. The con: Someone can grab it and stab you. Before packing heat or a hairpin, do a risk assessment to evaluate whether you're quick on the draw. I'm thin enough to be blown to the ground by a sneeze. An attacker could easily disarm me and slash me with my own blade. It'd be better to shout instead. If you do choose to carry a weapon, know how to use it when under pressure, and practice. Mace is not an option in several states including Wisconsin and Massachusetts, which restrict its possession. All that being said, most sexual assaults are committed by an acquaintance, so you're unlikely to have sharp keys in your fist if a date pins you down in the living room. You need other skills.

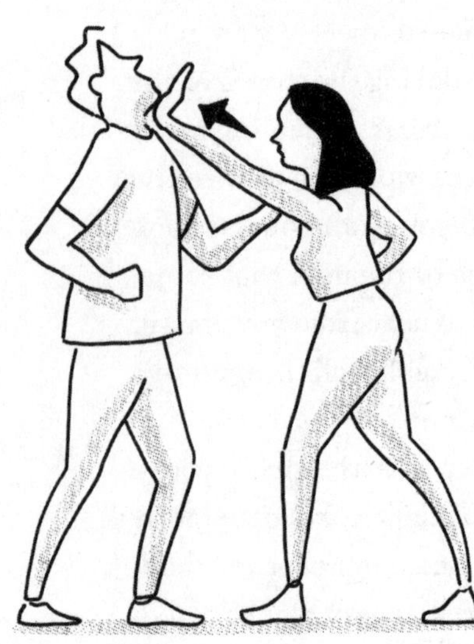

Becoming a Black Belt ninja requires years of schooling, and while martial arts can be a plus, it's worth training for more immediate results in terms of women's "self-defense." The techniques involved in such training are aimed at prevention, teaching women to be more assertive *before* the need to fight back arises. We also need to reset the way we use our voices and negotiating skills as a form of defense. Because we live in a society where our bodies are treated as objects, we can learn to move through the world differently by rethinking our potential strength and setting limits before we throw a jujitsu move or karate chop. It's also imperative to get comfortable enlisting others to intervene on your behalf, or to have friends nudge you to leave a party when you're too wasted for informed consent.

I endorse an effective national assertiveness program that's been around since the 1980s and requires just a few hours of training. It's called "model mugging," and I've incorporated it into my safety workshops, for all genders. As the name suggests, an instructor models what to do when mugged. You learn not only how to roll over when pinned down on a bed, but also to trust your instincts to leave a situation before things escalate and to use your voice as a deterrent, with loud shouts. Courses are offered all over the country through a nationwide organization called IMPACT, and some universities have signed on as well, under a program called Flip the Switch. Researchers at both Stanford University and the University of Windsor, in Canada, have found that the benefits of the course last for months if not years after it ends. (See Resources.) I took my first six-hour introductory class nearly ten years ago, and it became my favorite training exercise of all time. This is how it goes. Sixteen participants get to knee a pretend pervert in the goolies. We line up and run through drills where we variously stomp on sensitive bits, break holds, jab fingers into eyes, and pound privates. The method hits home that much of the human body is vulnerable, even that of a larger person. The aim is to throw the attacker off balance, not fight.

A well-aimed strike can win you valuable time to run, as your biggest weapons in such circumstances are getting some distance and calling attention with noise. The simpler you keep it, the better you'll remember it. All you need to do is stand firmly and swivel quickly with distracting shouts of "NO!" The stance resembles a boxer's, with the hands up and palms facing out.

The "perpetrator," an actor, wears a heavily padded suit and a helmet two feet high, so designed so that we can smack him without causing permanent damage. He doesn't look entirely human because of the gear, but his lunges replicate those in real-life situations. The scenarios vary: You may be reclining on a sofa or ambushed on the street or in an elevator. Everyone else watches as one participant after another plays victim, and when the perp strikes, so does she. She breaks free and wallops him so hard he reels back and falls. If a trainee pleads weakly, "Go away," the instructor makes her redo the exercise until she lets loose a banshee's "LEAVE ME ALONE!" Those standing on the sidelines hoot and cheer. Then it's on to the next volunteer, in what I would term a positive Me Too moment. When the instructor calls for more "victims," everyone waves hands, calling, "Me, too! Me, too!" We practice the moves again and again and again, until they become automatic, like riding a bicycle. But slamming a sleazebag is a lot more fun than riding a bicycle.

I strongly recommend the training for any woman, man, and child who has endured unwanted grinding, unsolicited advances, or violent assault. (See Resources.) The strategies are intended to help fend off a direct attack, but just practicing the yells alone can help you become more assertive when facing nonphysical harassment. By learning to use your voice and knowing that your body can serve as a weapon, you'll feel more empowered to verbally stand up to someone who is bothering you, as well as swing a good punch at the testes.

Shouting

WTF-- NO!
SICKO!
SHAME ON YOU!
HEY, LOOK AT THAT GUY!

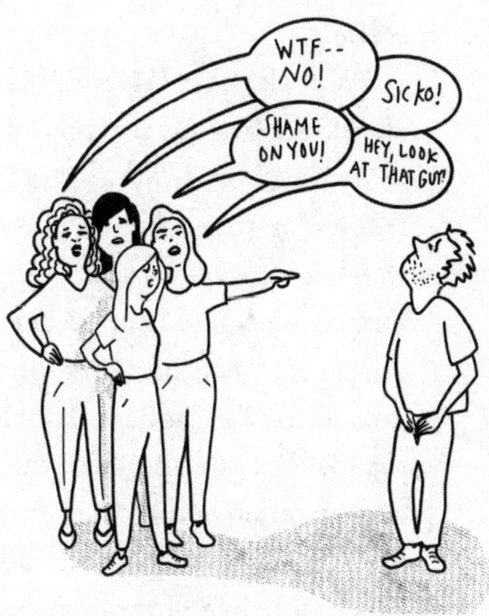

I am an extremely loud person, someone for whom hollering comes naturally. My whisper sounds like an ordinary individual's talking voice. I roar even when I'm not angry. I didn't realize my pitch deafened others until my mortified teenage son pointed it out. The last straw was when I yelled, "YOU WANT LUNCH?!" at one of his buddies who was at the house. After that, my kid writhed with dread every time a friend met me. His lasting discomfort convinced me to get my hearing tested. After sticking things in my ears and making me hold up my finger at shrill noises, the doctor pronounced nothing wrong. "You're just one of those overexcited people who lack self-awareness," he concluded. Thanks, Doc.

Despite having such a thunderous voice, for many years I had difficulty standing up for myself in public when threatened. I have no trouble bossing other people around inside a building, but something comes over me in an outdoor space. For a long time, I feared I was going to make a fool of myself for making a fuss over nothing. Many women share this self-doubting affliction. Often it's unclear if you're actually facing danger; lots of gray areas exist—until the assailant actually grabs you and sticks his hand over your mouth. Plus, women are brought up to be nice. This holds us back from making a well-deserved and potentially lifesaving scene.

Well, all those IMPACT classes have erased my reluctance about trusting my instincts and acting on them.

Aside from swatting techniques and bellowing "NO!," IMPACT also teaches us to enlist bystanders to intervene—*which is super important*. The trick is to identify a specific person and give him or her specific orders—"You, in the purple hat, call nine-one-one!" A vague "Help!" often does not suffice. Bystanders all look into their phones and secretly rejoice that the slimeball didn't target them. You shouldn't expect onlookers to step in and wrestle the person to the ground, as that could actually escalate the situation. But they can help embarrass or scare the harasser off.

I had a very satisfying experience revisiting this approach one sultry afternoon on the A train going from my house to the gym. A hyped man who acted like he was high on stimulants aggressively challenged everyone on the train to a fight. For some reason, he zeroed in on me, perhaps because I was the smallest and oldest person in the compartment. Meth Guy leaned over my seat and threatened to slit my throat. He had a powerful build that took up a lot of space. I am petite, and do not, so I could not wriggle away. As to be expected, fellow passengers remained happily distracted by their devices instead of coming to my aid. I elbowed the lady sitting next to me, but she pretended not to notice. So, I tried the "You, in the green jacket, call nine-one-one!" line. And it worked! The strapping man in the green jacket did even better than phone. He hauled Meth Guy off the train with the parting words, "You don't treat little old ladies like that!" I was tempted to holler, "Who are *you* calling an 'old lady,'" but that was enough confrontation for one day.

Street Smarts 101

You probably know all this, but I'll lay it out anyway. Avoid dark alleys and roads when alone. Don't walk with your face in your phone or with earbuds in. Make sure your cell phone is fully charged, and wear a rape whistle. Deploy peripheral vision at ATMs. Set the phone to emergency SOS. Make sure someone knows where you are if you're going to a high-crime area or on a lonely drive at night (or on a date with a stranger). The Find My Friends app comes in handy at such times. Plan routes ahead of time so you don't get lost, and stride with purpose, preferably in the middle of the street and against traffic. Yes, in the middle of oncoming traffic! That's another reason not to bury your face in your phone. You're less likely to be pulled into a building if you're in the road, and passing drivers will witness any manhandling by an assailant.

Extreme Techniques

A male safety trainer once advised that, as a last resort, pee, vomit, or defecate on yourself. I've never had the opportunity to try this out, but logic would have it that being soiled with someone else's bodily excretions would put an assailant off sex, or at least give him pause. I would imagine it's not easy to release bodily fluids on command, but you might just be scared enough to pull it off. Along similar lines, you could also tell the would-be attacker that you're menstruating, pregnant, and, by the way, have gonorrhea, syphilis, or are HIV-positive. Such conditions might disgust him, and the thought of contracting AIDS might even convince him to put on a condom. That could buy you time to stop the momentum and get you out of the situation—because, in the end, that's the ultimate goal here.

IF THE WORST HAPPENS

A proper sexual assault forensic exam by a medical professional enhances the chances of prosecuting an assailant. Using an at-home rape kit jeopardizes the case, however. Don't swab the semen and put it in a vial yourself. Legal experts caution that self-collected evidence will not be accepted in court. That's why so many sexual assault advocates and district attorneys have issued firm warnings against DIY kits. It's bad enough that women are not believed in so many instances; make sure that the evidence is obtained and stored through the proper channels. Aside from collecting semen, a licensed professional can document other signs, such as abrasions, bruises, and tears. So, if you've been attacked, head unshowered to a medical center, make a report, and have them do the exam for you. Hospitals have the added advantage of providing counseling by social workers, an important resource to help you through the crisis.

And: Tell someone. Now. Don't keep it bottled up. Don't blame yourself. It was not your fault. Talk to trusted friends or family. Seek professional help. If something terrible happened—and harassment and assault are terrible—you deserve support. No one should endure such things alone.

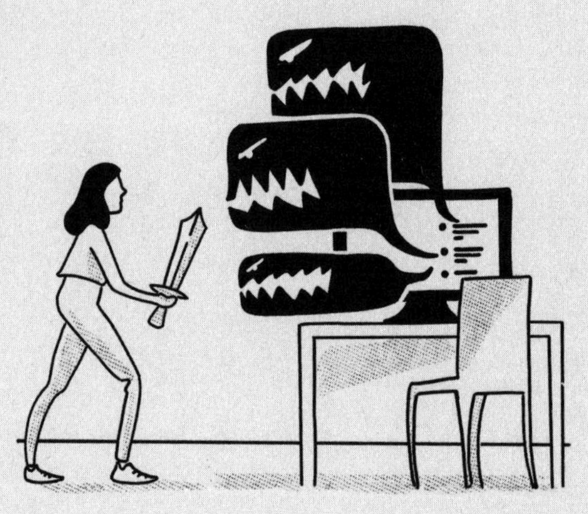

Chapter 10

ONLINE HARASSMENT AND STALKING

The internet isn't a nice place. Ugly, messy, hateful corners are increasingly bleeding through into the everyday. At a recent safety workshop, I met a woman journalist who had received threatening emails from a reader. Let's call her Sally, to protect her identity. The reader objected to Sally's articles about local politics and had posted furious comments. Journalists routinely get trolled on stories, so Sally did what she usually did: ignored it. After a while, the vitriol died down, so she figured it had blown over, as many of these cyberstorms do.

It hadn't.

A few months later, she advertised a garage sale on her Facebook page. She didn't think twice; people sell unwanted stuff that way all the time. Sally gathered old appliances and kitchenware, put a price tag on the items, and waited for neighbors to show up. As expected, people came—lots of neighbors and friends and a few acquaintances . . . and someone else.

You guessed it: the fuming reader. He had been cyberstalking Sally, and he showed up at her house as enraged as ever. Fearing he might be carrying a concealed weapon, Sally threatened to call 911 if he didn't leave. She informed everyone else present that he was a threat. Fortunately, this persuaded the surly man to leave the premises. But the incident was unsettling. He knew where she lived. He could come back another time, when there weren't witnesses.

This is why we need to think carefully about separating the personal and the professional online. We all have different spheres in our lives—work, home, socializing, parenting—whose borders are easily blurred thanks to our phones and the internet. The one thing we have control over is what we choose to post, especially pictures and our whereabouts. We can't control what Facebook shares with advertisers, or prevent governments from snooping into our cell phones and tracking where we've been at whatever times. Platforms such as Google and Facebook store a massive amount of data on users, such as geolocations and browsing habits, all of which has the potential to be abused. Cell phone providers and websites routinely sell our data to advertisers; that's why when you search booking sites for cheap hotels in San Francisco, you receive a raft of articles about Bay Area activities. So, unless we unplug entirely, we'll just have to make peace with that.

Government and corporate surveillance is intrusive, but shadowing is downright dangerous if perpetrated by a hostile individual who appears at a garage sale on the basis of personal information you've shared, like photos and your whereabouts.

Of course, we love social media. It brings us quasi-closer to long-lost friends. We can search! We can share! We can post! Some of us depend on Facebook and the like to publicize our work and gain clients. Social media provides a sense of belonging—and therein lies its curse. We trust "friends" or "friends of friends" because we "know" them. We are all part of the same network, and everyone is on Facebook, so it must be okay. But that's precisely the problem. *Everyone* is on social media. Facebook has about 2 billion accounts. Twitter claims about 140 million. Somewhere along the line, a vast number will be compromised, by fake accounts or hacking or slander. The very same anonymous and ubiquitous nature of the medium that broadens outreach also allows criminals and the malevolent to invade our privacy to wreak havoc. Malcontents can not only use online tools to trail us, but can also deploy tweets and fake accounts to spread venom or ruin our reputations. Anonymity gives them a cloak to say things they wouldn't dare utter to your face, and it saves them from having to see firsthand what their words do to you.

This online torment particularly tortures women, for whom the digital world is increasingly an unsafe space. According to the Pew Research Center, more than 40 percent of online users have experienced harassment, and it's women who are more likely to suffer the kind of severe hectoring that gets really personal, and sexual. We're called whores, bitches, slobs. We're threatened with rape, beatings, and death, or attacks on our families. We receive public shaming about our faces and bodies. While men are more likely to suffer intimidation because of their political views, women encounter sexualized forms of abuse at much higher rates. This is particularly true of women age eighteen to twenty-four, who are *more than three times* as likely to be sexually harassed online as men. (See Resources.) According to the Department of Justice, women comprise 75 percent of stalking and cyberstalking victims. Unwanted phone calls and messages were the most common aggravation, although about a third of victims reported that the offenders showed up in places without a legitimate reason or waited around for them, indoors or out. The internet helps the bad guys hunt you down.

All this constitutes cyber harassment, which is a grown-up term for the cyber bullying that takes place among teens. Cyber harassment involves repeated or severe targeting that can take various forms. Doxxing is when a malicious person uses the internet to publicly reveal online personal information—hence doxx, from "documents"—like a telephone number or email, for harassment or exposure purposes. Dogpiling is a coordinated attack by a group of online users via a barrage of threats, slurs, and insults. It's upsetting and can even lead to physical harm. Due to online heckling, many of my female colleagues have canceled accounts or changed profiles, or they self-censor what they post. Some went off social media entirely, and a few have moved homes. While cutting yourself off from the internet may seem safest—the lower the presence, the lower the chance of harassment—it's not realistic in our networked world. If you want to remain safe while connected, measures exist to lessen the risk. Without doubt, prevention is the most effective path. Once the abuse is out there, it becomes hard to remove.

EXPOSURE EXPOSES

A German woman I met in a workshop received offensive emails from a work contact. The messages escalated into physical threats: He published her address online, and strange men appeared at her apartment building, throwing rocks at her window and lurking about outside. She figured out that he'd probably located her through Facebook, or from doing a simple online search.

I invite you to take a closer look at your Facebook "friends." Do you really *know* all of them? At last count, I had 874 "friends," and to be honest, I haven't met most of them in person. I socialize with only about twenty of them. For me, Facebook is strictly about business networking. Decide what each of your platforms is for and manage your privacy settings and contacts accordingly. You're not going to see a picture of my cat, Henry. I don't post pictures of my family vacations. I like my vacations because that's what they are, vacating the real world with my son and husband, so sharing would be antithetical to the experience. I also don't want malicious people to know where I am, or even just that I'm not at home. Exercising discretion about what to share makes me less vulnerable and provides some insulation, as does using the highest security setting possible. That said, even if you've upgraded to the super-duper-highest-security private setting, which you should be, sometimes the accounts bounce you back to public. And whatever the setting, be wary about what's posted about you on any website, message board, blog, or social media platform. Do you use a discrete username for each platform? Username duplication can help a nasty follower stitch together a profile of your activities and likes. Don't post about places you frequent, like clubs or restaurants. A colleague who was being shadowed by a group of hostile men posted pictures of herself with her daughter at a pool where they liked to swim. If anyone wanted to harm her or her child, they knew just where to find them. Do you announce that you're about to leave for London for a weeklong trip? Do you link Instagram and Twitter accounts or sign into Spotify with your Facebook account? By doing so, you're giving a big platform much more access to your life. Do you post any information on your page that could reveal your password or bank security questions or your location (pets' or kids' names, anniversary date)? Just publishing the obituary of a parent or a wedding announcement can make it easier for someone to find personal details. Your full name, birth date, email, home address, and telephone number provide a gold mine to doxxers who can post your personal information without consent.

Security-savvy journalists are deliberate about what they share in public spaces, and dedicate separate accounts for social, financial, and professional matters. If they use Twitter for work, they restrict photos of kids to other venues. They also use dummy laptops when they travel. We'd all benefit from doing this.

SELF-SEARCHING

I do an exercise in training that always shoots up the blood pressure. Participants try to find out as much as they can about each other, based solely on what's available online. As a starting point, all they have is the name of the other person. Try it. Google yourself and see what comes up. While you're at it, check out online databases like AnyWho, Whitepages.com, Spokeo, and Intelius. I gagged the first time I did this. With a few clicks of the mouse, anyone can find out your birth date, address, email, name of firstborn, and more. The cost of your house, your marital status, and your arrest history are all out there, too. Who your parents are, where you've worked, everywhere you've lived—that's why none of those particulars should be in passwords. All a villain needs to do is figure out your passwords, and if you use the same one for several accounts, they'll be on their way to obtaining your Social Security number and bank account details. For that reason alone, you shouldn't use the same username for various platforms. You'll make it harder for someone to glean insight into your tastes and habits if you have different usernames for, let's say, online chat rooms and Facebook.

Fortunately, data mining sites often post erroneous information. For some reason, some list me as living in Brooklyn. (I have never lived in Brooklyn, but don't tell!) One site claims I'm a resident of Arizona. If only! I'd pay less in taxes and have warmer winters. I'm fine with these misperceptions precisely because they're wrong. I'd worry if any information were correct. If yours is, request to remove a listing on these directories. Keep in mind that aggregators such as Spokeo access publicly available information from other sources, so the data may still appear elsewhere, and the directories may well repost data after it's been removed. It's a pain, but worthwhile to check periodically. I prefer to pay someone to do it for me. For a little over one hundred dollars a year, the DeleteMe service of the online privacy company Abine will remove listings every three months. (See Resources.)

I also suggest accessing Google's "Me on the Web" tool. Set it up for personal info like your address, telephone number, and name, and it will let you know when any of that compromising stuff pops up online. This method saves you from having to google yourself every day to see if someone is writing bad things about you or pretending to be you. What's more, it allows you to remove offending content.

HAIL TO THE BURNER PHONE

I mentioned burners in chapter 3 ("Bring It On—Travel"). They serve a great purpose when you're not on the road, too. The drug dealers on my street use these babies to avoid detection by eavesdropping law enforcement, although they speak so loudly that the head of the NYPD could hear them from miles away. My son, who to my knowledge is not a drug dealer, calls burners "Mom dinosaur phones" because they don't have "smart" features like cameras and games. Dinosaurs or not, burners are brilliant because their users can't be tracked and generally don't need to give out identifying information when buying one. Some cost as little as $20, so

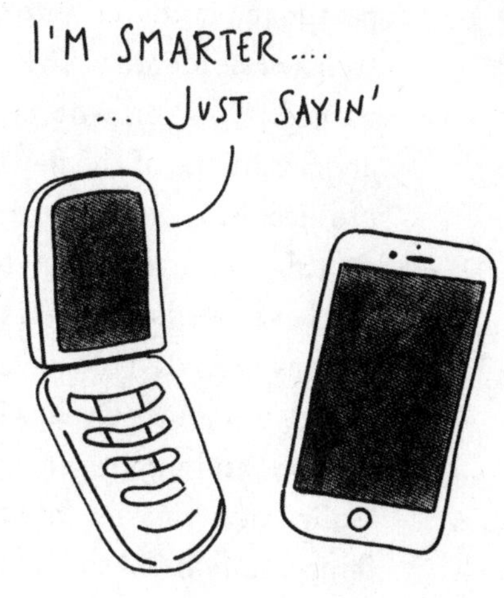

you can throw them away when you're done. Compare that to the $850 price tag of a smartphone. The drawback, of course, is that you can't hail an Uber or stream podcasts with burners. I'm all for buying a smartphone, but share its number with a small group of trusted friends and family only, and use the burner phone for public contacts.

For other communications, my security guru, who understands how these things work but for fairly obvious security reasons asked me not to reveal her name, suggests setting up a permanent unlisted phone number via Google Voice, which allows you to place and receive calls from anywhere. Or check out Twilio. When your app gets a text, Twilio asks how you'd like to respond and includes data about the incoming message, such as the contents and the phone number it was sent from. Or set up a profile on MySudo, which breaks the link between online accounts and the personal information associated with them. If one account gets hacked, the rest don't.

HOW TO SPOT A TROLL

Trolls often use the anonymity of the Web to post incredibly cruel messages. Generally, their social media presence lacks personal photos or information, in order to obscure the troll's true identity. They are probably not using their real names. A person who posted nasty comments on myriad articles in one of the newspapers I contribute to didn't have profiles on LinkedIn or Facebook, which made me suspect that she, if it even was a she, was hiding behind a fake name. The best defense against trolls is to report and block. If the trolling is related to work, ask your employer to respond and report the abuse. Otherwise, ignore the jerks. They crave attention, and might get even more abusive if you respond. I realize this is easier said than done, but don't give in to the temptation to tell them off.

Standard operating procedure is to report abuse to the providing platform. You should do this in case the platform is logging volumes of complaints about any one account. But don't expect much. What with their millions of followers, Facebook and Twitter say they lack sufficient resources to investigate every grievance. That generally leaves you to block harassers yourself. Blocking is a good first step, but here's where it gets tricky. Yes, both companies have mechanisms to prevent harassers from seeing your account or messaging you anymore; they won't be able to find you when they search your name. But fiends can, of course, create a new account and start up all over again. For this reason, on Twitter at least, I recommend that you mute rather than block. Muting prevents the offensive comments from appearing, without the aggressor knowing that you can't read them. They'll hurl abuse into a void without realizing that you won't read it. Now, that's sweet revenge! The one downside is that muting them doesn't make them go away, so you might want to enlist a trusted person to keep an eye on what the trolls are saying, in case they issue death threats.

Another course of action is to assemble a team to respond to the harasser on your behalf. Ask all your friends and coworkers to report the abuse to the platform and circulate screenshots as well as the responses they get.

REPORT THREATS AND STALKERS

Vicious comments are upsetting. They're annoying and unsettling. Doxxing, however, can get really dangerous if people use the information that has been posted without your permission to hunt you down in person. Abuse in the form of comments can feel obnoxious or even sinister, but the kind of response you take in the event of a true physical threat is more serious. A lot of women I meet are loath to alert authorities. They don't want to make a fuss in case they're exaggerating the danger. Or they are reluctant to go to the police because of past experience, or because they know law enforcement is not on their side. Whether you go to the police is a personal decision, but ask yourself: Do I feel unsafe? Do I worry about the security of my kids, my partner, and my parents? Never, ever ignore a threat. If an antagonistic or aggressive individual threatens to harm you or shows up at your house, parking garage, office, or anywhere—make a report to the police or even the FBI's Internet Crime Complaint Center. A report to authorities aids the building of a legal case. Go with a trusted ally in case you don't have full confidence in the police, which is perfectly understandable. Often cops are dismissive, or may not even know that the abuse is illegal in your state. Calmly but firmly give them logs of incidents (dates and times; screenshots of texts, chats, and emails; recordings of telephone calls). Share any identifying information such as the harasser's physical description and license plate number. The law is on your side. The Federal Violence Against Women Act includes provisions against electronic stalking, and all states have some form of antistalking legislation on the books.

If the stalker is harassing you by phone, install the CallerSmart app, which helps you identify mystery numbers and avoid unwanted calls and texts. (See Resources.) Change your phone number to an unlisted one, or install a virtual phone number through Google Voice.

Physical stalking is incredibly unsettling. If you haven't already, disable geo-location settings so that the stalker can't hunt you down in person. Vary habits such as walking routes and appointment times, if possible. Tell coworkers, friends, and family not to give out personal information to the stalker or post anything about your movements or status online.

Avoid being alone, and look over your shoulder when walking outside. If you're being followed, inform the stalker clearly and directly that they should stop, and then cease any contact. That's for the police. Duck into a store or bank where there are lots of people and tell the cashier and customers present what's happening. Usually someone will go out and confront the offender, and offer to call the cops. Bolster security at home, such as installing window locks and bars, security cameras, and an alarm. If you're freaked out, consider leaving town for a short while.

REVENGE PORN

Your risk assessment before getting into bed with anyone should include the possibility that the hot charmer you're infatuated with might turn out to be a jerk and post pictures of your intimate parts online without your permission. The obvious way to combat revenge porn is not to let anyone (not even you) take sexy pictures of you that could fall into the wrong hands.

If you're reading this with a deep red face, take solace in the fact that you're not alone. According to the Data and Society Research Institute, revenge porn has afflicted as many as ten million Americans. (See Resources.) More than forty-five states have outlawed it, but don't invest much hope in prosecuting on the grounds of stalking or harassment, because the websites that publish the images have probably never met the victims, or have reposted the shots from elsewhere.

If you've taken and shared racy selfies—which the vast majority of photos used in revenge porn are—do not despair. This will sound crazy, but listen. By law, any picture you snap yourself belongs to you, whether it's risqué or not. You can claim copyright, which gives you, the artiste, legal grounds to demand that search engines and websites take the darned thing down. Register the images with the Library of Congress. Yes, lodge those racy videos with the U.S. government. You don't need a lawyer for the copyright registration, but I suggest you get legal help to prepare the cease-and-desist case. It feels creepy knowing that some clerk may see your T and A, but the picture is already out there. The poor sod is just one more person, and is there to help.

Chapter 11

DODGE THE HACK—ELECTRONIC SECURITY

One of my star trainees, Alex, nailed nearly everything in our safety workshop. She immediately grasped how to deliver a precise kick to an assailant's groin, and could fell a ripped pugilist quicker than you can scream "Muhammad Ali!" She tied a tourniquet like an EMT paramedic and could drag a body twice her weight. Let's not even talk about her risk assessments for sinister assignments. The CIA would be lucky to have Alex as an undercover agent. Confrontations don't faze her; she could probably negotiate her way out of a mugging.

The cyber safety workshop, however, tripped her up. As the instructor showed the trainees how to use encryption software, Alex's mind grew fuzzy, and just the word *encryption* set her pulse racing. During the sessions where students installed and practiced using sophisticated encryption tools, her mind turned to mud; she couldn't focus.

"The encryption stuff seems to be a language I don't speak," she told me with considerable frustration. "It's in its own universe."

I get it. I'm with you, Alex. Tell me there's an earthquake, and I've got you covered. Cross fire? I can handle it. Follow me! But going to the Apple Store freaks me out. I am probably one of the biggest cyberphobics in my profession. Cyberphobia is an irrational fear of computers, and boy, am I afflicted. The salespeople speak gibberish, and they're way too cool to be patient with me. I don't like machines in general, and get easily frustrated when they malfunction or when I can't figure out how they work, which is a lot of the time. I fear I won't be able to master ever-evolving software and worry that my colleagues will make fun of me as I struggle. While my computer anxiety borders on the pathological, I see severe discomfort all the time in cybersecurity workshops.

Alex is fairly typical. Few journalists easily master how to scramble their emails and envelop videos with protective software. As a result, data distress discourages many of us from mastering the sophisticated encryption tools that can actually make us safer. But let this serve as inspiration. If I can overcome such a mental obstacle, anyone can.

It's incumbent on us to feel comfortable with intimidating technology because short of unplugging completely, we face escalating risks to our privacy, personal information, and identity. New technology is constantly being tested and adopted and applied, and we have to keep up with it. The unpleasant reality is that we live in a world where our most important data can be robbed or sold onward, as we saw with the 2017 Equifax breach, with Facebook's sharing of user data with third parties, and with the constant flow of software viruses that replicate harm to our computer files. As inconvenient and time-consuming as taking precautions may be, and they are a royal pain, we need to shift our overreliance on technology from sharing to protection. We don't want scammers to empty our bank accounts or run up $25,000 in purchases on our Mastercard, or an airline to share our facial features for recognition purposes with third parties. Think about it this way: You lock your car door; you should padlock your internet dealings.

When contemplating how to renegotiate a relationship with IT, privacy and data protection should be your lodestars. The former involves the government or companies invading your personal space and using something, like your habits and voice, to spy on you or to sell this information onward. The latter involves unfriendly parties hacking into your accounts in order to steal your identity or data. This particularly worries journalists because we deal with sensitive information and confidential sources, but it should also worry anyone who has a bank account, Social Security number, and credit cards—that is, all of us. It's important to step back and think about what information is most precious and needs to be protected. Always ask yourself: Who might want my stuff? How might they get it? How can I foil them? Depending on what lurks in your life, the answer to the first question might be a petty criminal, the National Security Agency, or your craven ex. The answer to the next two questions involves learning how hackers or governments spy on your business and then taking action against such an eventuality. For that, I recommend taking a course and staying abreast of the latest protective software. What I have found is that hands-on training and repeated practice under the tutelage of a patient instructor (with a stress on *patient*) works best for gaining competency. My brain clouds when I go on search engines to obtain instructions on how this or that works. I need a human being who can speak and point at my screen and lead me through the process, over and over again.

Case in point: I recently googled "troubleshooting PGP," for info on Pretty Good Privacy, a super-cool encryption tool favored by investigative journalists. One entry went like this:

Q. Are PGP 2.6.x, PGP 5.x and higher, and GNU Privacy Guard interoperable?

A: By and large, all PGP 2.x, 5.x, and GPGs can interoperate if:

Only RSA keys are used, of at most 2048 bits length,
MD5 is used as hash algorithm
IDEA is used for the symmetrical algorithm.

For GNU Privacy Guard, this usually means that you need to add the IDEA module as detailed in the gpg faqRSA support is included by default as of version 1.0.3. Newer GPG versions include a—pgp2 option to restrict the output to things that PGP 2.x understands.

I had no idea what this meant. I'll bet you don't, either. But I'll bet your fifteen-year-old niece who learned how to code in middle school can decipher these words, or knows someone who can. Get her to walk you through the installation process. Ask her to practice sending encrypted emails back and forth with you. Or maybe her tech teacher, or a grad student in computer science, wouldn't mind tutoring an adult like you. Or you could consult two excellent cybersecurity outfits that organize events around the world to make us all digitally adept citizens, the Electronic Frontier Foundation and CryptoParty. Organize your book group, or a circle of trusted friends who won't laugh at your lack of savvy, to hold a tech gathering with their experts. The Electronic Frontier Foundation, an international digital rights group, publishes information about tools and holds events around the world. It fields queries and gives updates about vulnerabilities. You can request a speaker. Or attend one of the free events on digital protection held by the global movement CryptoParty. Discussion subjects can include encrypted communication, avoiding being tracked while browsing the Web, and general security advice regarding computers and smartphones. You can attend one of its many get-togethers or organize your own through the website. As with first aid, I suggest taking a deep dive into practicing the knowledge so that it becomes as automatic as bandaging a wound. (See Resources.)

Hackers and digital eavesdroppers gain access to your dirty, or clean, secrets in many nefarious ways. They will use spyware, viruses, and keystroke logging (aka keyboard capturing). They will figure out easy passwords and look over your shoulder on the train when you sign into your phone. I'll discuss fixes for all these points of vulnerability, but first let's talk about correcting bad habits. Behavior modification is as important as using protective software.

RESET THE MIND-SET

When my safety class takes bathroom breaks during digital training sessions, I swoop around the room and collect the cell phones and laptops participants have left behind on their desks. They don't think twice about leaving them unattended in the room for a few minutes, and I capitalize on that. I pluck the memory cards from the cameras. I might even send text messages to myself from the devices, for added fun. Once everyone returns from the recess, they generally don't realize for at least a few minutes that their devices are missing. Then they panic.

I don't do this to be hateful. I do it to illustrate a powerful lesson about letting down one's guard. It hits home that when it comes to the machines that guard our secrets (or really anything), you can't trust anyone, anywhere. You can install all the elaborate software you want to encrypt your data and manage your passwords, but without the simplest precautions, rogues can abscond with your stuff. Most of us are lulled into a false sense of security because we haven't thought through the vulnerabilities. And these weaknesses are often at the most basic level.

Those of us in the safety world call it digital hygiene. Think of it as cleaning house, rather than molars. You probably wouldn't leave the front door of your house open. Why would you step away from your iPhone? It contains everything precious to you—contacts, credit card details, that photo of the dog when he was just a puppy. That should remain private. All a malicious sod has to figure out are your passwords, and as we discussed in the previous chapter, if you use the same one for several accounts, they're on their way to obtaining your Social Security and bank account numbers.

Granted, I work in a profession where survival hinges on cyber caution. If a reporter's sensitive information gets out, sources can be skewered on social media, thrown in jail, or even chopped up with hacksaws. Reporters, too, can be jailed or chopped up. We have to be vigilant against cyber eavesdroppers, snooping governments, corrupt politicians, drug traffickers, organized crime, and petty criminals. So many different parties want access to our files, data, confidential sources, and social media accounts. They want to blackmail us by finding out what we're up to or with whom we're sleeping. Or they'll do something unsavory with our information. We're under constant threat. We cross borders with sensitive photos and documents in our computers and phones. Repressive governments track our movements and emails to identify whistleblowers and leakers. An opportunistic terrorist might steal your money. That happened to Matthew Schrier, a freelance photographer who was kidnapped by Syrian rebels in 2012. His captors figured that while they had him, they might as well demand his passwords and PINs to drain his bank account. He eventually went free, much poorer.

While reporters are particularly vulnerable to cyber break-ins and eavesdroppers, ordinary citizens face risk, too. So do cities. In 2019, at least 113 governments and agencies, including Baltimore and Albany, fell victim to cyberattacks, which scrambled their data with unbreakable encryption and shut them out of email systems and payment platforms. (See Resources.) Elsewhere, millions of Americans have been victims of identity theft at home, touched by the breaches at Target or Equifax, to name two. While traveling, businesspeople and tourists need to protect their personal and financial data as well, especially in high-crime and oppressive countries. Yet, even knowing this, we fail to back up files or change passwords regularly because it's a pain in the neck. Plenty of people use the same password for thirteen different accounts, or write passwords down on a sticky note tacked to their monitor. Others leave memory sticks lying around on their desks. Life becomes safer and, dare I say, easier with a healthy dose of internet paranoia, however. Yes, digital safety is a pain, inconvenient, and mind-boggling. But if you want to protect your money and emails from hackers and crazy ex-boyfriends, it's worth taking protective steps. Aside from being sinister, being hacked can destroy your life.

VIVA ANALOG!

Back when I started my career, 1,050 years ago, we did fine with rotary phones and telex and typewriters. Voice recorders ran on tape, and cameras required film and something called darkrooms. We went to the bank to deposit checks. We wrote notes with pen and paper and then threw them away when we were finished. Navigation meant you had to know where you were going or chart it out on a physical map. Then everything shifted to digital, and for a while we thought that the digital stuff was safer. It's retrievable. You can't just lose or misplace it in the cloud. You can typically recover whatever it is these days—but so can other people who want to get their hands on it.

In my book, analog still wins the day. Invest in a fireproof safe at home to store paper records and other valuable files. As uncomfortable as we all are writing down personal details and passwords, a well-hidden little black book stored in the safe is often more secure.

Having read about my training session, hopefully you won't leave your iPhone on your desk at the office. Don't leave devices switched on continually, either. Turn them off except when they're actually needed. Aside from saving on battery power, and sparing yourself from annoying social media alerts—I don't need to know that you're stuck in an airport, or that your kid just got a trophy—you'll limit exposure to hacking. Every minute online increases the possibility that someone could barge in. While you're at it, get a screen protector that prevents Joe Schmo from looking over your shoulder at Starbucks. The following are other tangible ways we can stop compromising our digital safety:

PASSWORDS AND TWO-STEP VERIFICATION

All safety measures can fail without airtight passwords that are updated periodically. I know, I know. It's a total drag to reset each one every two weeks, as the experts recommend. But even every six months would make a difference. Choose difficult-to-crack passwords, and never duplicate them among multiple accounts. Birthdays and kids' names, "password," and "abc123" are no-nos because they are so easy to figure out. Avoid "fuckyou," which apparently is another popular password. To get the hackers off track, the passwords should be at least sixteen characters long. That's right, sixteen. And don't share them with anyone, except one point person who will know how to close down your accounts in case you're hacked (or dead). Insert punctuation marks and numbers to break up the words. If you find that confusing, do so at the start or end of the password. I like sentences or movie titles because they're harder for a hacker to figure out. A security whiz suggested I look around my kitchen and dream up a password based on random items in the room. That might lead to a password like "99basil,shears,Pierre,andknife!" Another trick: misspell the words or choose foreign ones written phonetically, words that no one would associate with you. For instance, if you loathe frogs, choose the Spanish word *rana* and then write it as "Ranna." (Since I'm mentioning frog/rana/ranna, obviously pick another word.) Avoid choosing something that might appear on your Facebook page, such as your alma mater or your parakeet's name.

This can get awfully confusing even if you're not changing passwords every two weeks. It goes without saying that you shouldn't store all the passwords on Google Docs, or on a piece of paper that's lying around for anyone to see. Someone could get ahold of them. That's why you'll want a password manager that does all the work for you. It generates unique sequences that no one could possibly figure out. What's more, it stores them all in a virtual vault that is encrypted and automatically inserts them when you log on to different sites. LastPass, 1Password, and KeePass figure among the offerings. *However*, you'll need a password to get into the vault itself, and I can't begin to tell you how many of my acquaintances forget this all-important code. That's where the fireproof safe comes in.

Another thing: Avoid "Save My Password" on browsers. If

they're stored on your computer, someone can log in when you're not looking.

Increasingly, financial institutions and businesses require two-factor authentication, which is supposed to protect you even if someone learns your password. It creates an extra layer of security by requiring you to verify your identity with a random code sent to your cell phone. Set it up for all accounts. But add a third tier of protection because, well, those clever devils in the hacking world have found a way around the two steps. This ruse is called SIM-jacking, and the way it works is that a scoundrel pretending to be you calls the provider to say you've lost your SIM card and need to reroute phone traffic to a new one. Once the pretender controls your phone number, they can hijack your social media and financial accounts. So, ask your provider to place a PIN on your phone account.

Security questions are gold mines for hackers who have gotten ahold of passwords. Often the true answers to security questions can be easily found on a Facebook profile or online. But you know what? You can lie! There's absolutely no reason to reveal the make of your first car, or Fluffy the cat's real name. A security-conscious friend once entered his mother's maiden name as "mud"; the system accepted it. How was it to know her name was really "Smith"? I find "mud" a tad harsh, being a mother, but you get the idea. Feel free to let the creative juices flow, as long as you remember what PIN you chose.

Triage Accounts

Now that you've set up the password defense, analyze your accounts and close any superfluous ones. The breaches at Equifax, among other companies, are to some extent beyond our control because the firms store our personal information as soon as we do a transaction. But we lay ourselves open to identity fraud by overexposure. The more credit cards and accounts you have, the greater the chances that someone can steal your Social Security number and impersonate you. Many of us checked our credit scores after the Equifax disaster and then we promptly stopped doing it. Make that a regular practice every three months.

While we're talking about spring cleaning, weed out apps periodically. And don't give third-party apps access by signing in with Facebook, Twitter, or Gmail.

ROTTEN PHISH

Not to be confused with the Vermont rock band, this ruse involves "fishermen" who send out lines with bait into the vast sea of the internet, hoping to hook victims with an innocuous email address line like "Hi, Judith!" The email looks like it's from a legit organization, but don't be fooled. It lures you to a link on a fake website where you're asked to share your credit card or bank or password details to address some fictitious payment issue. I hate this scam because I've fallen for it, as have countless millions of other unfortunates. We're too trusting. Don't click on SMS links from senders you don't know; delete them immediately. Don't answer inbound calls from numbers you don't know. Don't respond to links that say you owe money to the IRS, PayPal, or any other company. Don't respond to emails that claim you've won money. Install apps only from the app store on your phone, not from individual websites.

While you're at it, keep an eye on the elderly, who are particularly vulnerable. Scammers love to target old people, who often lose track of their financial affairs as time grinds on. My late mother, for example, asked me to check her credit after Equifax identified her as possibly compromised. I was staggered to discover that she had nearly ten credit cards for various stores. This was a woman, mind you, who was confined to a wheelchair and hadn't gone shopping for years. She wore the same comfortable clothes each week and could barely read books anymore, so the Lands' End and Amazon accounts should have been canceled. She didn't recall that she had all these cards. While you're at it, make sure Grandma has all the latest antivirus software installed, which you may have to run for her, and that she knows not to open messages from strangers. That goes for you, too. (You've heard it before, but I'm going to say it again.)

ONLINE BANKING

Don't lodge security codes and credit card numbers on your phone in an unencrypted note that anyone can see. Refrain from doing online banking in internet cafés, hotels, or the airport. Use only trusted financial hardware and software, like Apple Pay. It's designed to protect financial data and keep it in one highly guarded space. Venmo is safe as long as you're making a payment to someone you know and trust. Furthermore, never trust a site with your personal information that isn't https-encrypted.

What is encryption? you may ask. Basically, it scrambles letters so that a third party cannot decipher the message. Say you write, "The dog needs a walk—badly." The message looks to an eavesdropper something like this: *6FG/wgryQ1AQ//X7RZgF+r1Uwwpf.* That's encryption. Many applications do this automatically, so you may have installed this technological wonder without being aware. Check.

A caveat. Encryption technology is safe only as long as it's safe. That's the problem with digital "protections." Their effectiveness ceases when some hacker figures out how to bust the system, and you learn the system is compromised only after the fact. Therefore, knowing all these fancy applications and programs lends a certain false sense of security. For that reason, it's important to stay abreast of any breaches and patches issued to resolve them. Install updates when they come out, as they may address vulnerabilities or other problems. Tech giants are constantly looking for vulnerabilities in their systems and working to patch them. To ascertain if a data breach has affected your emails, and set up alerts going forward, go to https://haveibeenpwned.com. (Not to be confused with the haveibeenpawned.com on Amazon. Remember not to type in the *a*.) (See Resources.) If you're running a blog or a website, consider switching to a content management system like WordPress, and let them take care of updates for you.

THE DANGERS OF AIRPORTS, HOTELS, AND INTERNET CAFÉS

I know. We've all signed on in a café or hotel business center, or while waiting for a train. Free public Wi-Fi is convenient. You've got to message someone immediately or pay a bill. But some bad guy may be watching you type, eyeballing the passwords and keystrokes you're entering. Equally dangerous, you forget to log out, which enables the next person sitting in front of the screen to capture your sensitive data. Or maybe the internet café owner has installed spyware that gains access to passwords and other personal info by tracking keystrokes. Remember to close the browser and delete your browsing history before leaving any public computer.

To make life easier, set up your own portable VPN router, which is wireless and fits in the pocket. Don't get a free or cheap one; it might track and sell your info. It's worth shelling out the sixty dollars (or more) for a trusted VPN like TunnelBear or Vypr. It allows you to safely surf the Web from your car, hotel, restaurant, or out on the street. A VPN, which stands for "virtual private network," hides your communications by scrambling data and routing it through a private server, thereby obscuring your location and computer. Think of the private server as a pipeline that no one can crack. VPNs are excellent for online banking and accessing the office computer from a laptop while on the road. Or for watching HBO overseas! Acquaintances use them in China in order to access Google, Facebook, and other sites that are blocked or censored by authorities. Having said that, be aware of the risks of using a VPN in China, and a handful of other countries, like Russia and Iran where they could get you into trouble.

Let's say you've already signed on to networks and want to cleanse your laptop of them. Go to System Preferences (or Control Panel) on your computer, and then Network. It will list every network you've been on, from free Wi-Fi at Starbucks to ones that had a password at a hotel. Sometimes, if you've opened your computer at a store with free Wi-Fi, you will get online automatically—and that's a portal for hackers. Hit Delete to get rid of the record. Alternatively, so that you don't automatically sign on to the free networks while trying to delete them, uncheck "Automatically join this network." That's less of a risk.

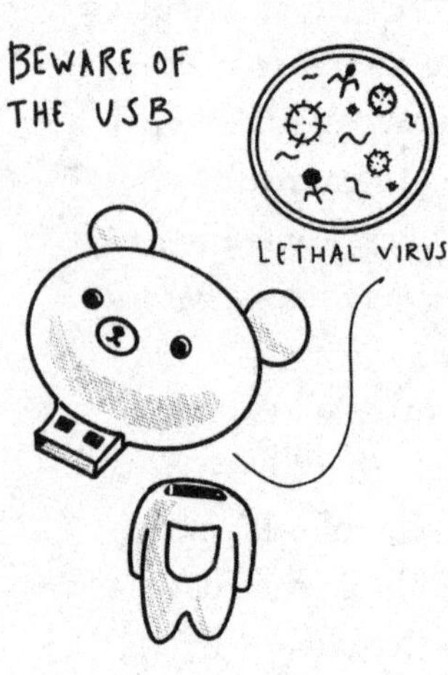

Finally, we need to talk about USB flash drive sticks. They're small! They fit in a wallet! They back up lots of data and important documents! They're great for business presentations! And they are among the most common vehicles for spreading malware, including at an internet café. When sticking one in your laptop, you could pick up viruses from another computer. So, think of flash sticks like soiled tissues. Throw them away once they've been used. Don't accept one from another person. Also, to share presentations online, opt for tools like Google Drive, which also saves you from worrying where you've put the darned stick.

Signal

A messaging app with end-to-end encryption, Signal can be installed on Android, iOS, and desktops. It's easy to use—and free! Security folks prefer it to WhatsApp and iMessage because it's open source. That means you don't have to take the company's word that the software is secure. Being encrypted, messages would appear as nonsense should authorities subpoena the company in charge. What's more, the service can be configured so that a message automatically disappears. And one doesn't need usernames or passwords because mobile numbers are how contacts identify you. I've heard complaints about occasional glitches and users like me who don't answer their phones when a Signal call rings. (Both parties have to be on it to use it.) Friends who want to get ahold of me through Signal will text to notify me that I should check my Signal.

Steady, though. In some countries, such as Venezuela, Signal sends up red flags that you have something to hide. Before traveling, research to see if WhatsApp, which also has end-to-end encryption on messages, is a safer option. Yet keep in mind that Facebook owns WhatsApp, and it has intrusive priorities, like tracking who's talking to whom and when and where. Another concern, which mostly affects women: Some of us wish Signal didn't require a telephone number, which means handing out one's personal phone number to potential contacts and the public at large, which can lead to abuse. For that reason, women might want to look at Wire instead, which requires a username and password, and offers nearly the same features.

CHILDPROOFING . . . AGAINST CHILDREN

Let's make one thing clear. I cherish my son more than anything. I didn't know I was the maternal type until age forty-three, when I gave birth to him. All of a sudden, I realized that I would inhale all the tear gas in Paris to save him. No, all the tear gas in the entire world. I would climb into razor wire and stand in front of a barreling armored tank to protect my boy. I would throw out every piece of advice in this book if it meant rescuing him from peril.

That said, I won't let him near my computer. We parents are rightly worried about protecting the kids from internet ogres (porn, perverts, and drug dealers), but we should be equally worried about protecting ourselves from them. Not knowing any better (or not thinking it through enough), our children import viruses by clicking on seemingly innocent games or ads. Here's a cautionary tale. There once was a sixth-grader named Brian. (His name has been changed to protect his identity, as hopefully he has grown up to be an upstanding citizen who drinks responsibly, respects women, and never drives through red lights.) Brian liked to browse porn instead of doing his algebra homework. He shared links with a friend who was curious about sex. Unbeknownst to the boys, the porn was infected with malware that allowed the friend's parents' computer to be hacked. Mom and Dad were not pleased.

Even if your kid doesn't have friends who surf porn, regularly delete Spam emails that land in your inbox. This prevents children from accidentally, or intentionally, opening links that contain bugs. Regular deleting provides the added satisfaction of getting rid of annoying unsolicited advertisements from companies that provide stuff you'd never want to buy.

TRICKS FOR ELUDING FACIAL AND VOICE RECOGNITION

Movie star Greta Garbo was ahead of her time when she donned a low-brimmed hat and enormous sunglasses and apocryphally declared, "I vant to be alone." (Or "I vant to be left alone." The exact wording has come under debate.) Her getup would have helped foil the facial recognition technology that's threatening our privacy today. From Walmart to schools, technology that can analyze one's features and face shape can potentially violate an individual's rights. I don't know about you, but I don't like the idea that a hotel or fast-food chain has my mug entered into a system to identify me for God knows what purpose. Short of walking around with masks or balaclavas, which are likely to arouse suspicion on any day but Halloween, modern-day Garbos have options for confusing the cameras.

First, big sunglasses and surgical masks go a long way toward hiding sections of your face. If you want to go all out, wear hairdos or makeup à la Kiss, which distort the face's symmetry. The fashion site CV Dazzle offers some snazzy examples. The designs draw inspiration from a type of World War I naval camouflage inspired by Cubism. I'm particularly taken with a blue-and-platinum-black coif that hangs over half the face, with a makeup smear on the opposite cheek. You can also trick the cameras by wearing someone else's face on a T-shirt or mask. I'd personally opt for a Groucho Marx mask with plastic nose and bushy eyebrows, even though it would make me look riduculous. However, bear in mind that some states ban the donning of disguises in banks or to evade the police, though what that means is open to interpretation.

I'm waiting for Reflectacles to hit the market. (At the time of press, they were advertised but not available just yet.) The developers of these special eyeglasses claim they can trick infrared cameras into not seeing the face. Ready when you are!

Smart Speakers

Smart speakers like Apple's Siri and Amazon's Alexa work as recording devices that can be remotely accessed via the internet, which creates the potential for abuse. Next time you say "Okay, Google," mute the microphone after hearing the answer and delete interactions that have already been recorded.

IF I HAD A HAMMER

You've decided to get rid of the old computer. Before you dump old faithful in the trash or donate it to charity, destroy its hard drive, which contains all the sensitive files you don't want anyone else to get their hands on. Don't just hit Delete for files. Permanently get rid of them—with a hammer or another tool like a drill. That's right. Smash the bugger to bits. Pretend it's the boss you always hated! YouTube offers many tutorials on this destructive and highly satisfying activity. Put simply, make sure you haven't left a CD or USB stick in the computer, so as to leave no secret behind. Back up the really valuable stuff, like photos and music. Then disconnect the cables to avoid electrical shock and unscrew the computer casing (not as easy as this sounds) and look for a magnetic disk. Each model is different inside, so check the operating manual or ask a fourteen-year-old geek to rummage about.

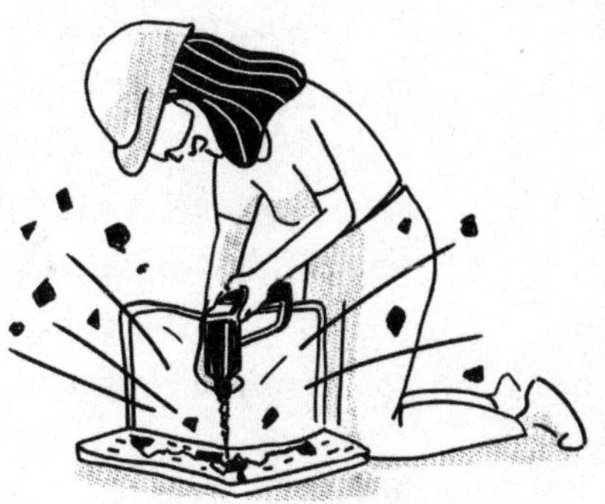

Wrap the disk in a cloth, put on goggles, crank Led Zeppelin to the highest volume, and whack away. Discard the shards separately to prevent the Russian spy lurking around the trash can from puzzling it back together. Contrary to urban legend, soaking a disk in bleach won't erase data, so if you lack a hammer, and feel in the mood for drama, blow up the hard drive with dynamite or shoot it with high-caliber bullets. Incinerating it will also do the trick, but this is a job for a licensed data destruction company, not the backyard barbecue.

Safety can be fun!

NINJA TOOLS (FOR SPIES, THE PARANOID, AND THE REST OF US)

These tools are not for the fainthearted. I can demystify these marvels only to a certain extent. They're for computer systems engineers and hard-core investigators, politicians, human rights activists, and businesspeople who fear digital spying by governments or competitors. Basically, anyone who needs to communicate sensitive data free from surveillance.

Before you start installing any of the tools I describe here, double-check the legality in the country where you're traveling. Also consider that encryption tools can send up a red flag that you want to hide something. In a country like Turkey, certain protective software can get you detained on spying or antiterrorism charges, even if you're simply trying to keep your nude photos private. Another thing: The truly safety-aware use a combination of various tools. They make phone calls via Signal, browse on Tor, and send messages via PGP. Alternative tools are out there, but these are the most commonly deployed by the cyber savvy.

PGP

PGP stands for Pretty Good Privacy, and it's pretty hard for ordinary users to master it. Still, this software has reigned supreme among whistleblowers and investigative reporters for thirty years, allowing them to communicate privately without being surveilled. Its popularity exploded after Edward Snowden used a similar method to share his NSA revelations with journalists in 2013. Put simply, PGP involves complex keys that allow two parties to scramble and unscramble secret messages. If the ploy works properly, no one else can decipher the messages.

PGP looks really neat in the documentary about Snowden, *Citizenfour,* when the letters are typed on the movie screen. Sounds good, right? No! My trainees whimper when it comes to the PGP lecture because, as I've said, it's devilishly problematic. Just installing it and doing practice runs will cause headaches, if not existential dread. Contemplate devoting the effort to it only if you're really, really going to use it. Otherwise, the headache's just not worth it.

Tor

Tor stands for "The Onion Router." Unfortunately, it's not as funny as *The Onion* satirical news site. Think of an onion, with many layers to peel away. The core is your information, which is protected by many layers of subterfuge. Journalists love Tor because (a) it's free, and (b) it prevents others from learning their location or browsing habits by hiding the IP address where a message originates. A remote server sees only the proxy's information. I don't have enough technical prowess to explain *how* Tor does this, but you can read about it yourself on www.torproject.org. Tor is often called "the people's VPN" because seven thousand volunteer computers participate in the project to keep your data safe. Tor is easier to master than PGP—really, *anything* is, except flying a space rocket—although it's notoriously slow. Users report that messages get lost occasionally, but if they are technical ninnies like me, they may be using it incorrectly. Ironically, the U.S. Office of Naval Research funded the initial research, and now many Tor customers, including criminals, use this VPN to avoid American government surveillance. You can run Tor automatically through Tails, an operating system installed on a USB stick or a DVD that doesn't leave a trace on a computer. Edward Snowden apparently liked this one, too. Check the website tails.boum.org to fully glean how it works.

CONFUSED?

Yup. Computer security is complex. But trust me, it gets easier with time, so it's best to set aside a couple of days to dive into the wonders of the digital safety world. Hacking is preventable, and a few small changes can make a big difference in securing your life.

Chapter 12

MENTAL ARMOR—EMOTIONAL RESILIENCE

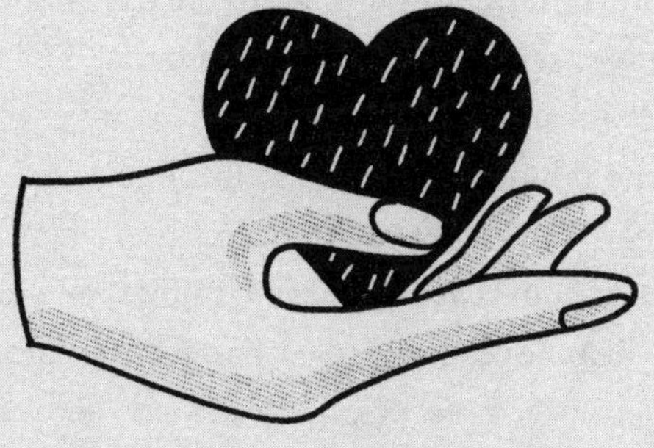

Okay, so you've followed all the tips so far. You've calculated all the risks. You've gathered the material you need and have an exit strategy. You now know to stay at the edge of crowds, deflect annoying harassers, and secure your electronic communications. You've packed an emergency kit and dived under a table during earthquakes. You've checked for exits at big gatherings.

Even so, the dreaded day arrives—as they do, despite the best planning. You're at a concert or sports event, and a mass shooter attacks the crowd, killing dozens of spectators around you—an event like the Ariana Grande concert in England in 2017, or the Las Vegas massacre that same year, or the Boston Marathon bombing in 2013, or the shootings at Florida's Pulse nightclub in 2016, or September 11 in 2001. An unexpected, devastating attack.

Or the cyclone floodwaters reach your house, and they've risen by four feet. You've got to get out of there fast. Or the earthquake sirens sound as the earth rumbles, and rumbles again. Or you hear loud shooting—bang bang bang bang bang bang—at an office reception. Or armed men are beating up the protesters around you at a march. Or maybe cyber abuse and doxxing have eroded your sense of safety, and you feel threatened just returning home at night.

Understandably, you feel panicked. Your heart beats way too fast, and you want to jump out of your skin. Your chest constricts, and you feel like you can't breathe. Instead of calling 911 or shouting for aid, you feel paralyzed. But you need to keep moving. Channel your imaginary yoga guru. Inhale through the nose, holding for a few counts. Exhale through the mouth. Repeat five times. Inhale. Hold. Exhale. In through the nose. Out through the mouth. Visualize a happy outcome to the crisis. You're going to swim to safety with the dog under your arm. The kids are safe at Grandma's. The insurance company will replace the roof that just blew away.

You can't control the active shooter roaming the halls or the earthquake that just shook the bookcase off the wall. But you can control your response. Breathing calms your system. There's a scientific reason for this. Deep breathing sends oxygen to the brain, which helps maintain focus. In a study of mice, researchers at Stanford University found that the nerves in the brain that control breathing are linked to the arousal center. Apparently, we're like mice when hyper-aroused by stress hormones. Once you feel more clearheaded, concentrate on a specific, immediate task (such as finding a barrier to hide behind or barricading the windows or powering up the generator). That will keep your mind off contemplating what might spin out of control. This is the one time you don't want to dwell on the worst-case scenario. This is not the moment, either, to question your abilities or fast-forward to a dire outcome. Take action and power ahead.

THE AFTERMATH

Being prepared, you ducked the gunshot/explosion, remained upright during the stampede to the exits, or managed to tie a few tourniquets on the wounded. Or you got the family to shelter. You stayed quiet in the closet until law enforcement shot the shooter. You managed to stay calm. Well done!

Even if you survived any of these, or a terrifying run at a protest, or the mess in your house after a hurricane, it doesn't end when you flush all the tear gas out of your eyes or clean up the mold. You also need to look at how you feel. Just because you have lived through an experience physically doesn't mean you're done with your survival mechanism. You can't possibly control everything by anticipating every outcome—accepting this is essential to emotional resilience—but you can anticipate that extreme scenarios will give you a serious fight-or-flight jolt. Let it move through your body and be aware that it's happening. Like grief, stress has cycles that are deeply individual and take time to work through. The following tips are geared toward traumatic events, but they're also useful for the ordinary stresses that stem from a toxic conversation with a boss or burnout or the death of a loved one.

SELF-CARE

Establish Routines

Trauma begins in the body. During a stressful event, the body is flooded with cortisol and adrenaline, which give you more energy, and it takes time to restore balance afterward. Most people feel anxious in the days and weeks afterward. You might have trouble sleeping, and crowds may make you anxious. A backfiring car sends you hugging the pavement, and you feel overwhelmingly sad at random moments. It's hard to focus on work. That's a standard response to an extraordinary event, and it's important to regain a sense of control. These unsettling feelings will subside for many people, but will continue for others. Both reactions, short- and long-term distress, are completely normal responses. When they persist and interfere with life, there are tactics for enhancing emotional resiliency to better cope and mitigating emotionally toxic reactions. These can include specialized trauma therapy and a series of healthy habits to boost management of moods before and during trying times.

Grounding routines with regular meals and bedtimes help enormously to keep physical arousal low. Set schedules provide structure after an emergency that's rattled one's feeling of safety. Have rituals to mark the end of each day with something pleasant. Put on music, ride a bike, or revisit an image you find especially soothing. (For me, it's a particular hike in Arizona—with no rattlesnakes.) A friend who was taken hostage described how establishing times for exercise and washing in her small cell helped her regain a sense of power, however slim. She felt she could control one thing. (She also asserted herself by demanding better-quality food from her captors, but I'm not recommending you do that with housemates.) Consider what anchors and relaxes you—something like going for a swim, meditating, or gardening. If you, like me, have trouble sitting still even without a stressful event, then by all means don't go to a beach and ruminate. Even if you like sitting still, don't go to the beach during jellyfish season. I did that once during the war in Mozambique and got stung all over, which made it hard to sleep and eat, actions that we have established assist recovery. I also stayed in the sun too long and got terribly burned. Really bad times two.

I personally prefer to remain busy—swimming, talking, dancing, talking, hiking, talking, and, well, talking. This frenetic activity can drive my husband and son crazy, but, hey, a girl's gotta heal. And, well, I know my family will stick with me no matter what—or I hope they will. When the guys tire of my whirling dervish pursuits, I seek out furry animals that provide unconditional love and won't bite. It has to be a species that remains quiet as I pour out my woes. Our pet chinchilla was a terrible listener; he ran in his exercise wheel without a shred of sympathy. I could barely hear myself speak above the squeaky treadmill. A friend acquired a therapy horse, which provided her great joy until it kicked her in the leg; she had to wear a brace for ages. I recommend the more dependable dog. It will do anything you want if provided with the right bone. Unlike friends, it won't say things like "I know how you feel" when it has no idea. The dog will not pretend to understand you, except when you take out the leash to go outside. Apropos, dog walking provides exercise and lends structure to the day. You have to get up in the morning, or it will poop in the kitchen. And what could be more altruistic than picking up poop in the street?

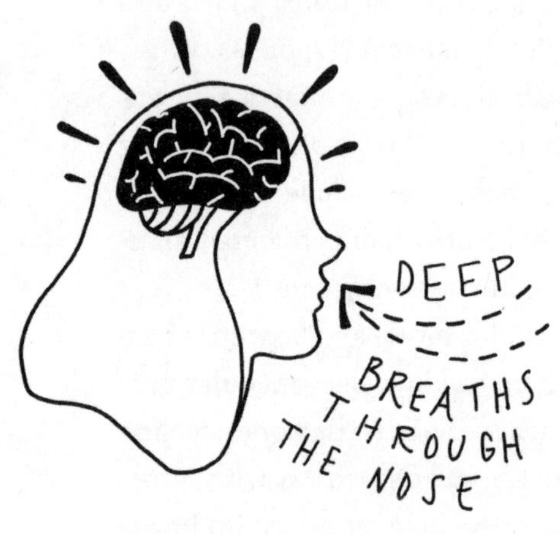

I also clean the house like a fury when under stress. Scraping stove grease to roaring music like the Clash provides an immense sense of satisfaction, in my book. And the scouring wins brownie points from everyone else in the house (checks the altruism box). Spread the happiness around!

Social Glue

Psychologists say the one thing most associated with emotional resilience is social connection and support. No way around it: Isolation hampers recovery, and positive relationships do the reverse. It could be a close friend, an acquaintance with whom you feel comfortable, a support group of others who survived the event, or—and this is really important—a mental health practitioner. It has to be the right people, of course: cheerful and kind ones who make you feel worthwhile. Steer clear of fake sympathizers who ask in that lowered, funereal voice, "How *are* you?" Equally problematic: Sometimes the people closest to you may be the worst confidants precisely *because* they care so deeply about you. They're rattled to see you agitated, and then *they* stay up all night worrying about you, which in turn makes you feel guilty. You stop reaching out in order to avoid upsetting them, which then causes more alienation. I sometimes find that a more detached person makes the best listener in emotionally fraught situations. As mentioned before, many high-stress professions offer counseling or buddy systems. More informally, I have a circle of work comrades who keep an eye on one another's emotional temperature and intervene without being intrusive. We check in periodically and offer a home-cooked meal if someone seems to be struggling through a tough period. Our circle resembles a book group, except that we discuss nightmares instead of novels and don't critique one another's dreams. Generally, communities pull together after a tragedy, and you might actually find comfort in talking to strangers struggling with similar feelings rather than relatives or friends who don't really understand. Look for support groups that have arisen following traumatic events such as 9/11, and contact leading psychological associations that can help locate specialists who'll accept your insurance. Ask friends, your health insurance provider, or the family doctor for recommendations. (See Resources for a list of organizations.)

Also consider altruism. Nothing beats doing something nice for others. The other person appreciates the gesture, and you feel good about yourself. It's a win-win. Helping someone more miserable than you also puts things in perspective and gets you out of your own head. Visit a lonely relative. Babysit the neighbors' kids. Volunteer a few hours for a cause you believe in (or used to believe in before the world seemed like such a hopeless place).

Catching Zs is highly associated with emotional resilience, and it's crucial for memory consolidation and metabolizing difficult experiences. Being exhausted weakens your resistance. I realize that getting a sound night of rest is challenging when nightmares keep you up. However, it helps to have a sleep plan that involves regular bedtimes. Put away devices/screens an hour before lying down, and don't be available 24/7 to friends or colleagues. There's nothing wrong with asking the doctor

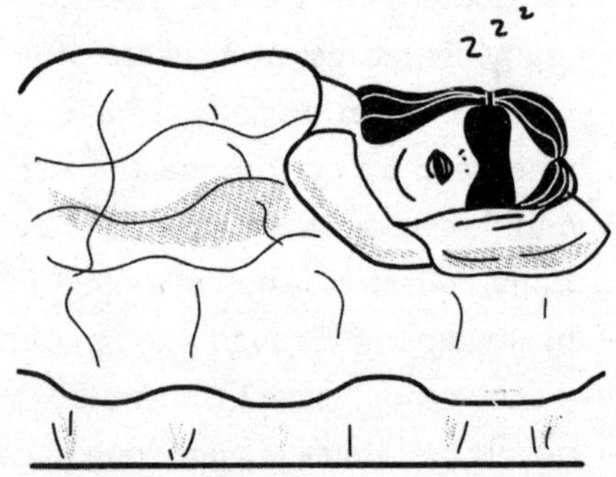

for prescription sleep aids to get through a crisis, but make sure they're not addictive pills of a quantity that will create a whole new set of issues.

Exercise

A good workout provides a healthier approach to dealing with stress than gobbling Xanax. Regular exercise is associated with resilience in the face of trauma exposure. Aerobic activities like swimming, dancing, and running are associated with controlling breathing and stress—the sort of thing where you get lost in the rhythm and empty the mind of bad thoughts. Exercise also dilutes the body of adrenaline and cortisol, the hormones associated with the fight-or-flight stress response. It will probably help you sleep better, too.

Food

Staying fed and hydrated helps with a sense of control, and organizing a regular meal plan is as important as juicing up your cell phone. You wouldn't let your iPhone battery run out; same with stomach fuel. Stress often manifests first with head- or bellyaches. A loss of appetite is my early warning signal that something's off, as I normally shove food into my mouth every couple of hours. It's important not to skip nutritious meals when you're feeling vulnerable. Eat properly and indulge in comfort dishes. My go-tos are melted cheese and ice cream (not together, although I once tried a delicious ice cream in Peru that was like frozen cheesecake). For some reason, milk products console me; I'm sure Freud would have a field day analyzing why. Whatever food group works for you, go for it. That said, don't go overboard guzzling three pints of mascarpone gelato a day. Weight gain doesn't help the self-image when you're feeling down, nor does rushing to the hospital with pancreatitis. Don't forgo healthy stuff like vegetables and fruits, which according to some neuroscientists help with resiliency. I've heard people who are not neuroscientists claim that various foods affect their moods positively, including wolfberries (aka goji berries) and fenugreek seeds. I have never ingested a wolfberry or a fenugreek seed, but any unprocessed item that's rich in minerals and vitamins can't hurt brain function. (See Resources.)

Humor

According to the neurologist Viktor Frankl, humor was one of the "soul's weapons" in the fight for preservation in the Nazi death camps he survived. Humor more than anything else, he explained, "can afford an aloofness and an ability to rise above any situation." (See Resources.) I couldn't agree more. There's nothing like a sense of the absurd to pierce the dread. Humor permits a bit of distancing. It's a way to connect with others and allows for perspective. Don't be taken aback if you hear others poke fun at what terrifies them the most. While dark humor may appear offensive to outsiders (or even insiders, for that matter), rendering horror ridiculous takes away its emotional power. Ever spend time after hours with surgeons, emergency responders, war correspondents, soldiers, firemen, or cops? Listen to their ghoulish repartee. They make tasteless jokes about bodies, blood, and gore. (Here's one I heard in Ukraine: "How do kids from Chernobyl count to one hundred? With their fingers.") Soviet citizens told jokes about the Stalinist purges that rounded up friends and other citizens. And prisoners of the Nazi concentration camps made cracks to keep up their spirits.

Gallows humor as a coping mechanism has appeared in nearly every conflict zone I've been to, all over the world. One example jumps out from some colleagues who spend each day facing possible murder. A couple of years ago, I conducted a grim training session for female journalists in Vera Cruz, one of Mexico's most vicious places. The topic was ethical coverage of sexual violence, always a downer for women for whom rape is an occupational hazard. At that time, Mexican newspapers printed grisly photographs of mutilated bodies on their front pages. The gratuitous images desensitized and traumatized readers, and served as propaganda for the drug cartel that killed the victims. I wanted to open a discussion on the media's responsibility. A female human rights lawyer and I stood at the front of a room and slogged through a slide show of images to make our point. Slide one: piles of bodies stacked at a massacre site. Two: a corpse with her head chopped off. Three: a naked body with a noose around its neck. One by one, we discussed the societal impact of seeing such images. Faces grew somber as we dissected each one. Oddly, no one left the room, but no one was saying much, either. They just stared morosely at the pictures. Uh-oh. This wasn't going well. The co-trainer and I shot looks at each other. Time to wrap it up. We showed one last photo, of a defaced torso on a bed. "What is wrong with this picture?" I asked, for the last time.

Silence. More silence. Then someone piped up. "It's out of focus, that's what's wrong." The room convulsed into raucous laughter. It was like opening a sluice gate. They couldn't stop guffawing. When we went for lunch, people joked that the shredded beef in the tacos belonged in the slide show.

Now, I'm not suggesting that you make morbid fun for the

sake of it. Far from it. Only that you consider the potential of comedic relief, refined or otherwise, to cope with emotional intensity. Watch silly rom-coms or cartoons. Binge on *Monty Python*. See stand-up shows. Scientific research shows that laughing is a stress reliever. It brings more oxygen into the body and can strengthen the immune system. Besides lightening the mood, you might live longer.

Om

Practice meditative pursuits like yoga and mindfulness, which keep arousal low and allow you to observe yourself. Try sitting quietly in a spiritual place. I'm not observant religiously, but I find houses of worship of any type soothing, particularly when no one is talking. There's something timeless about spirituality, and statues of martyred saints remind me that things could be a lot worse. Seek out other recreation that plants positive imagery—music, gardening, art museums, nature walks. All these pastimes have restorative healing powers. Start a journal. Ever wonder why so many war correspondents write memoirs? A narrative has a beginning, a middle, and most important, an end. Writing down an experience can aid self-observation and give you a sense of control.

PTSD

Sometimes, though, what you feel is something that going for a run or eating greens won't fix. Some people just aren't very reactive after a tragic or frightening event. Many people, of course, suffer for a few weeks, and some relive the shock for a short period of time. Yet, for others, as time goes on, the unease deepens, rather than lightens as you hoped it would. You feel guilty for surviving and can't enjoy parties. The panic attacks grow more frequent. One day, you drive by the attack site and . . . BAM! For a terrifying moment you're transported back to that appalling day. You conjure up the screams and the mangled flesh. When you go to bed, the fear and images return in nightmares. You think you're going crazy. You start avoiding friends. They don't understand how you feel. The world is a terrible place, and you feel so damned alone. And you ask, What the hell is happening to me?

What's happening is likely PTSD. People throw the term around loosely; just the other day, I overheard a college student complain that he'd gotten PTSD after eating cafeteria food. I'm sorry, that's not PTSD. That's just grumbling about dorm living. Get off the meal plan and learn to cook. True PTSD, or posttraumatic stress disorder, can occur following a violent and terrifying event. Being jittery and quicker to anger and having intrusive memories, nightmares, and flashbacks comprise one silo of reactions; another includes numbing and avoidance of interactions that might trigger reminders. Some people may have insomnia, or sleep too much. They may lose their appetite or overeat. Invariably, their worldview grows dark. People can experience just one side of these reactions, and suffer a lot, but not get a PTSD diagnosis. And there are lots of responses that have elements of PTSD but are more manageable. But a diagnosis includes a four-sided whipsaw of avoidance, reliving the events, negative thoughts, and hyperarousal.

PTSD is diagnosed as lasting for at least a month after the event, and it can resurface years later. (See Resources.)

Soldiers can get it. So can cops, EMT workers, and survivors of disasters and sexual assaults. Events like war, muggings, torture, rape, car accidents, school shootings, hurricanes, and wildfires can bring it on. Maybe a third of war correspondents have had it. According to the National Center for PTSD, 7 to 8 percent of Americans will experience PTSD at some point; the percentage is higher for women. It's far from universal, however, and plenty of people survive traumatic events without experiencing lingering emotional distress. True, PTSD can be debilitating and persistent if left untreated. And as we've seen with veterans returning from Afghanistan and survivors of the Parkland school massacre, it can lead to suicide. Women are twice as likely as men to develop PTSD symptoms (more on that later), but we are just as easily treated as men. And PTSD *can* be treated.

PTSD is a relatively recently classified disorder, which means that the science of care is still evolving. In the old days, it was called shell shock or combat fatigue. Those in Vietnam referred to the thousand-mile stare of soldiers who had seen too much horror. Only in 1980 did the American Psychiatric Association enter PTSD into its *Diagnostic and Statistical Manual of Mental Disorders*. Since then, professionals such as EMTs, firemen, and human rights activists have recognized the risk, and newsrooms are slowly embracing mitigation efforts. When I started out reporting from conflict zones, we all pretended we weren't having flashbacks or sobbing at night after returning home. *What, forty corpses? Ha! No big deal. We're not sissies.* Of course the threats and the exposure to violence affected us. Now journalism organizations are installing hotlines to specialized shrinks, and buddy systems whereby reporters who cover the cop or international beat watch one another for distress. The average civilian impacted by a stadium bombing or raped by a date doesn't necessarily have a professional cadre equipped to handle the psychological fallout, but if you feel left on your own, support groups and networks exist to help you through the crisis. (See Resources.)

Scientists don't know why some people develop PTSD and others do not. But repeated and extended exposure to violence seems to present major risks. War and sexual assault seem to be major triggers. This might explain why women are diagnosed at a higher rate than men: we are more likely to experience interpersonal violence. Some experts believe the data are skewed because women are more likely to seek help. Other scientists suspect that it has to do with brain wiring—though, so far, few studies can really distinguish between male and female responses.

Whatever the causes, here's what happens to someone who suffers from PTSD. The sounds, smells, and snapshots of a traumatic event embed themselves in the brain. You might, for instance, vividly recall the smell of burning tires, the screech, the crunch, the fumes, even a particular nervous shout after a car accident. That's because beneath the frontal lobe is the amygdala, the part of the brain primed for survival. Senses awaken, blood rushes to the muscles, and you breathe quicker as oxygen races to the lungs. If the threat is severe enough, the body mobilizes for battle or flight. You become super alive in order to survive.

The problem with PTSD is that the amygdala fires long after the trauma, like a little smoke from the toaster tripping your fire alarm. You may be in safety afterward, but the mind and body don't settle down. They take too long to recalibrate, and lock into a turbo survival state. Memory can come in the form of a nightmare or a flashback about the frightening night you were assaulted, or heard gunfire, or nearly drowned. A screech—not from a wounded victim but, say, from a little kid in a grocery store hollering for candy—makes your mind and body react just as they did after the car crash. Psychologists call this state "anxious arousal," and it's an overwhelming emotional spin cycle. The numbing and avoidance that occur are just as important, and may in the long run be the more debilitating consequences, leading to social isolation and an inability to confront painful memories or routine stress. In short, PTSD mixes a cauldron of varied responses that make it difficult to function and seek inner peace.

Treatment

Seriously, if you've experienced trauma, these things can fester, and there's no shame in going to talk with a mental health professional. PTSD is fixable and effectively treated. Some people's PTSD goes into complete remission. Others learn to manage or mitigate their reactions, and to handle periodic recurrences. According to the Department of Veterans Affairs, more than half of people who have received trauma-focused psychotherapy will no longer meet the criteria for PTSD. And there's especially good news for women. While women are more likely to be diagnosed with PTSD, they respond to therapy and coping mechanisms just as well as men. Therapy can also work for those without diagnosable PTSD but for whom trauma reactions get in the way.

Much stigma surrounds seeking therapy, but seeing a counselor well versed in PTSD is for most people the best way to recover. You don't need long-term analysis to probe your childhood relationship with Mom (unless she was a terrorist who blew up schools), but simply a trained professional who understands why you're reacting the way you are and who knows what to ask and say to redirect your thinking. A colleague from the BBC likened PTSD therapy to vacuuming a dirty carpet. It's a psychic cleaning. Every time he felt stressed after an unsettling assignment, he'd make an appointment for counseling. Just a few sessions would do.

When looking for a qualified psychotherapist, consider the distinctive skills of a trauma specialist. To date, the treatments with the strongest evidence of success for PTSD in adults include cognitive behavioral therapies that aim to rewire the thinking away from negative attitudes and find ways to challenge unhelpful beliefs. Exposure-based treatments that confront difficult memories in a safe way can also work. Sometimes these methods are combined with antidepressants. Besides medication and psychotherapy, one can enhance one's emotional resiliency in order to better cope with and mitigate emotionally toxic reactions. The Dart Center for Journalism and Trauma has identified various self-care steps that can help manage this disturbing disorder. These commonsense tips have become the gold standard for newsrooms whose staff is exposed to violence, and they've proved valuable for the general public as well. Everyone's different, but the basic principles apply: Be good to yourself, and give it time.

DRINK AND SUBSTANCE ABUSE

If you're in a noxious work situation and you down a couple glasses of pinot to calm down at home, that's not great, but you don't necessarily have a drinking problem. Watch out, however, if you start emptying an entire bottle after an event that is more traumatic than an encounter with a passive-aggressive coworker. Substance abuse is particularly toxic for PTSD, and it increases the intensity and chances of developing it. What you shouldn't do under any circumstances is imbibe like my friends the war correspondents, for whom drinking is a form of social bonding. Journalists are notorious alcoholics, for which I blame Hemingway. The fêted auteur went to excessive lengths to celebrate drinking, and ever since, journalists who want to emulate his writing have seen a ruined liver as the benchmark. "I drink to make other people more interesting," Hemingway infamously proclaimed. Journalists think *they* become more interesting if they quaff obscene quantities of anything anyone else is drinking.

This is clearly an unhealthy way to deal with emotional strain after a mass shooting or losing your house to a hurricane. It goes without saying, but I'm saying it here, that drinking impairs judgment, interrupts sleep, and leads to more depression. You are more likely to get into car accidents or arguments, have unprotected sex, and send ill-advised texts to the boss.

You need help to manage what's going on in your life. Some doctors readily prescribe antidepressants or anti-anxiety medication to relieve anxiety. Be extremely wary of Xanax or any of the related benzodiazepine drugs such as

Valium and Ativan, which can be highly addictive; your body can build a tolerance for them quickly.

LET GO

Most important, let go. Accept that you're not invincible. Take each day at a time. Reacting to stress is human. Take care of yourself, talk and seek help. And as with everything else, be prepared to expect the unexpected. You're going to be okay.

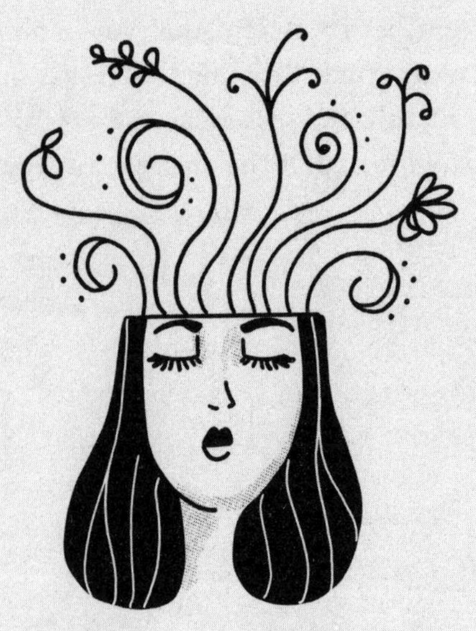

CONCLUSION

The people close to me joke that this book will blow up once you finish it. That's because trouble seems to dog me, even when I don't seek it out. I moved to Mexico after college and . . . bam! The peso collapsed. Then I went to London to cover the oil market. It, too, imploded. Thinking they were on to something, my bosses transferred me to the stock market desk. That was in 1987.

And so on. Plane crashes, street fights, a car bomb at Harrods in London, cholera outbreaks—stuff happens when Matloff comes to town.

In 1992, I went to Angola for the elections. The country restored peace only after I left. Same story in Russia—after I transferred there in the late 1990s, the Chechen war resumed. Oh, and the banks went under as well. Wanting a fresh start, I threw in the foreign correspondent towel and moved back to my hometown, New York City. A year later, September 11 occurred.

I'm not narcissistic enough to claim satanic responsibility for so many terrible events. But they do point to a truth. If you live long and travel wide, you'll likely run into bad stuff at some point. What's encouraging, though, is the resilience that comes along in the aftermath. Every crisis and emergency has made me wiser. They can make you stronger, too. A reserve of accumulated experience makes each calamity easier to face. I'm not saying that I grew callous, but I gained a thicker mental carapace and a store of knowledge.

With repetition comes aptitude and confidence. Each time you attend a demonstration, you'll remember how you kept to the sidelines at the last one. (You are going to follow that advice, right?) Once you've assembled your emergency kit for a storm, it's ready for the next big one. Living through any of the topics in this book prepares you for the others. It doesn't matter if we're talking about a shelter or a business trip or a grabby boss—the through line applies to everything: assess, plan, communicate, and survive.

The basic manual of information contained in this book is the first step; the next is practice. Seek out training in first aid, and in encryption software and rape prevention. Learn from the fire department how to escape a wildfire. Drills supervised by experienced professionals allow you to act out scenarios before they occur and divine how you might react. (Of course, I'm talking about exercises supervised by recognized experts and geared toward the appropriate age group.) Soldiers, journalists, and EMTs all do this for their work. We practice exercises, repetitively, until they become automatic. Nobody can predict how anyone will react in a crisis. You'd be surprised: Some of the highest-strung folks can be the calmest, and the normally self-contained can lose it. Going through the paces ahead of time will help you anticipate emotional triggers as well as perfect skills like dragging an injured body. You're less likely to become paralyzed, and you can jump into action quicker if you've done it before.

Watching someone do a task and then copying it with guided feedback is a sound path to overcoming fear, says Albert Bandura, a professor emeritus at Stanford University considered one of the luminaries of social cognitive theory. Bandura's tested this method on everyone from snake-phobics to combat veterans, and he's found that it helps an apprehensive person achieve a sense of control and even overcome trauma. Drills allow you to become creatively confident in crises. You develop muscle and mental memory and will feel more capable of improvising in fast-moving situations. Having been there before provides the knowledge for what to do next time. It allows you to act.

And keep consulting the tips in this book. Commit them to memory. Write them on sticky notes in the kitchen. Share them with your nieces and neighbors. And if the book blows up, don't worry. You'll know just what to do.

ACKNOWLEDGMENTS

As everyone knows, or ought to after reading this book, one shouldn't venture into dangerous situations alone. Also with books. You're holding *How to Drag a Body* thanks to several special individuals who took interest in this venture and ensured it got done.

The first bouquet goes to my dear agent, Joy Harris, who works magic to make ideas reality. I owe immeasurable debts to Alison MacKeen for brainstorming, and to Randi Epstein and Abby Ellin for cleaning up what resulted. Thanks for the edits, friendship, wit, and, dare I say, tequila.

Their efforts would have been in vain without the sparkling team at Harper Wave. I lavish appreciation on publisher Karen Rinaldi, who immediately grasped what I wanted to do—and then improved on it. Rave reviews, too, for Hannah Robinson, Rebecca Raskin, Jenna Dolan, Penny Makras, Laura Cole, Nikki Baldauf, and Sophia Lauriello.

Sharon Levy's cartoons captured the essence of the book. The woman can read minds and make their thoughts funnier. Love that llama in the basement!

I relied on the generosity of colleagues for insights into obscure matters like severed fingers. Bruce Shapiro, Elana Newman, Harlo Holmes, and Dr. Chris Tedeschi all agreed to critique sections of the book and caught some real bloopers. Thanks, folks! Tina Susman recounted cautionary tales from her spellbinding life. Sawyer Alberi taught me everything I know about dragging bodies, as well as stuffing chickens. Karen Chasen and Shep demonstrated how to knee a rapist. The world is a better place for all the dedicated safety organizations that share such wisdom with the wider public. A shout out goes to the Dart Center on Journalism and Trauma, ACOS Alliance, Rory Peck Trust, James W. Foley Legacy Foundation, Freedom of the Press Foundation, PREPARE Inc., and Wilderness Medical Associates International. You're my s/heroes.

The Logan Nonfiction Fellowship at the Carey Institute for Global Good provided a quiet haven for this noisy writer.

Now for the family. I dedicate this book to my mother, Hildy, who died before it was finished but delighted in hearing about the progress along the way. The woman was a model of managing risk, namely me, and she will always serve as my inspiration for resilience and unswerving love. Mom, you can RIP—I no longer do stupid things. Profound gratitude goes to the living—my sister, Susan, and my husband and son, John and Anton van Schaik. They don't complain when I withdraw into the writer's cave. They keep me fed, watered, steady, and amused. They claim it's no big deal, but believe me, it is. It doesn't get better than that.

RESOURCES

Chapter 2: The Basics

"Fluffernutter" has since come to hold a pornographic meaning in the adult entertainment industry, which might explain why parents in later generations took it off the lunch menu. Diehard fans of Fluff for sandwiches, not the triple-X variety, should not despair. National Fluffernutter Day is October 8, celebrated near the product's birthplace of Somerville, Massachusetts.

A chilling public service announcement produced by the March for Our Lives movement (https://www.thedrum.com/creative-works/project/mccann-ny-march-our-lives-generation-lockdown) outlines what to do in case of an active shooter. Consult a child psychologist to learn whether it's appropriate to share it with kids. In the video, called "Generation Lockdown," a schoolgirl sings a song taught by her teacher:

Lockdown, lockdown, let's all hide
Lock the doors and stay inside
Crouch down, don't make a sound
Don't cry or you'll be found.

Two leading experts hold forth on the psychological effects of lockdown drills on kids and the best practices thereof. One is Ken Trump, president of National School Safety and Security Services, a Cleveland consulting firm specializing in school security and emergency preparedness training (https://www.schoolsecurity.org). The other is Steven Schlozman, codirector of the Clay Center for Young Healthy Minds at Massachusetts General Hospital. The organization publishes an online educational resource (http://www.mghclaycenter.org/hot-topics/low-lockdown-drills/) that promotes and supports the mental, emotional, and behavioral well-being of children, teens, and young adults.

Chapter 3: Bring It On—Travel

The U.S. State Department website (https://travel.state.gov/content/travel/en/international-travel.html) offers a detailed checklist for before you go.

The International Electrotechnical Commission's "World Plugs" page can be found at www.iec.ch/worldplugs/.

The Centers for Disease Control and Prevention (https://wwwnc.cdc.gov/travel/destinations/list and https://www.cdc.gov/malaria/travelers/country_table/a.html) and the World Health Organization (https://www.who.int/topics/vaccines/en/) provide country-by-country rundowns of medical advisories and required and recommended vaccinations, as well as appropriate malaria prophylaxis for each locale. The CDC also provides information on special considerations for immune-compromised travelers or those with chronic medical conditions.

The U.S. State Department website (https://travel.state.gov/content/travel/en/international-travel.html) also advises travelers on commonly prescribed medications that are considered illicit or controlled substances abroad and therefore might be confiscated or lead to imprisonment after your arrival.

The outdoors store REI, the Red Cross, and various private outfits offer wilderness first aid courses around the country. A proper wilderness course lasts three days to a week.

The Iridium handheld satellite communicator costs about $350 plus a small monthly fee. It's helpful for natural disasters when ordinary cell networks crash.

Chapter 4: Just Plug It—Emergency First Aid

You can check your blood type at home with a kit (https://www.4yourtype.com/original-home-blood-typing-kit/).

Consult the Rhesus Negative organization's website (http://www.rhesusnegative.net/staynegative/rhesus-negative-friends-and-organizations-worldwide/) for a list of groups and resources worldwide.

First aid training can be found through the Red Cross and the National Safety Council. As mentioned earlier, I recommend a wilderness safety course, which will take you beyond the let's-pound-the-chest CPR. Because of its intense and comprehensive nature, you emerge capable of stabilizing a leg fracture or a neck injury.

The Stop the Bleed movement (https://stopthebleed.org/) offers kits and training that are lifesaving in active shooter situations as well as car accidents.

Various online resources train people to respond to opioid emergencies by administering naloxone (brand name: Narcan), the antidote to overdoses. Check out www.getnaloxonenow.org and www.naloxoneinfo.org/run-program/training-tools.

Chapter 5: Run! Protests, Bombs, and Shooters

Home Depot offers a selection of respirator masks in its Safety Equipment department and publishes a handy buyer's guide online (https://www.homedepot.com/c/ab/best-safety-equipment-for-painting/9ba683603be9fa5395fab900591e2ab).

Protest laws vary by state and city (https://civilrights.findlaw.com/enforcing-your-civil-rights/protest-laws-by-state.html).

Hit rates for police officers (i.e., measures of their accuracy with firearms) are surprisingly low (https://www.ajc.com/blog/get-schooled/gunfights-trained-officers-have-percent-hit-rate-yet-want-arm-teachers/mDBlhDtV6Na4wJVpeu58cM/).

Chapter 6: Do I Stay or Do I Go? Natural Disasters

The National Centers for Environmental Information publishes data and reports on disasters (https://www.ncdc.noaa.gov). The government's National Weather Service (https://www.weather.gov/) puts out alerts, updates, and tips for every conceivable form of bad weather.

The World Bank (http://www.worldbank.org/en/news/feature/2013/12/12/improving-women-disasters) and the United Nations Development Programme (https://www.undp.org/content/dam/undp/library/crisis%20prevention/disaster/7Disaster%20

Risk%20Reduction%20-%20Gender.pdf) have both issued sobering reports about gender and disasters.

The many products mentioned in this chapter, including models of hand-cranked NOAA weather radios, can be ordered online. Home Depot offers a helpful guide on the various respirator masks on the market (https://www.homedepot.com/c/ab/types-of-respirator-masks/9ba683603be9fa5395fab907a681adb).

The outdoors store REI gives a good rundown of the various types of avalanche transceivers (https://www.rei.com/learn/expert-advice/avalanche-transceiver.html). Many models are advertised online.

Chapter 7: Gimme Shelter—Hunkering Down When Disaster Strikes

A variety of LED headlamps, surge protectors, SAD lamps, and generators can be found at Home Depot or online.

Satellite telephones can be rented or bought. Leading brands are Inmarsat, Globalstar, and Iridium Satellite.

Chapter 8: Drinking

Moderation is fine. Excess isn't. Consult www.aa.org.

Women who drink excessively are more likely than men to suffer damage to the liver, heart, and brain. Alcohol abuse can hurt fetuses and have a negative effect on fertility and menstrual cycles. Consult the CDC Fact Sheets at https://www.cdc.gov/alcohol/fact-sheets/womens-health.htm.

M. Mohler-Kuo, G. W. Dowdall, M. Koss, and H. Wechsler, "Correlates of Rape While Intoxicated in a National Sample of College Women," *Journal of Studies on Alcohol* 65, no. 1 (2004): 37–45.

Chapter 9: #MeToo and Rape

Hollaback!, an international organization operating in twenty-five countries, offers strategies and resources for combating harassment (https://www.ihollaback.org/cornell-international-survey-on-street-harassment/). The website cites the Cornell study I mention in this chapter.

To find a state-by-state list of restrictions on pepper spray, go to https://www.pepper-spray-store.com/pages/states.

In 1990, a Stanford University team published a study on forty-three women who had taken model mugging training in the San Francisco area (https://modelmugging.org/journal-of-personality-and-social-psychology/). It found that six months after the course ended, the women felt freer to use public transportation and to go out at night. They were less anxious walking down the street and asserting themselves with forceful men. Further compelling research was conducted over the past decade by social psychologist Charlene Senn, from the University of Windsor, in Canada (https://charlenesenn.ca/eaaa/).

The Rape, Abuse, and Incest National Network, or RAINN (https://www.rainn.org), is the largest anti–sexual assault organization in the United States. It offers free and confidential services to survivors of assault, including a 24-hour toll-free hotline.

IMPACT has chapters all over the United States and holds assertiveness workshops at schools, colleges, studios, and private venues (http://www.impactselfdefense.org/). (No, I do not hold shares, in case you're wondering.)

The national working women's organization 9to5 (www.9to5.org) offers fact sheets and advice on combating sexual harassment in the workplace. To reach the helpline, call 1-800-522-0925, or email @9to5.org.

The American Association of University Women aims to promote gender equality through education, advocacy, and research. Its website provides many resources, including a legal guide to workplace sexual harassment (http://www.search-elnk.net/search/?q=http%3A//https//www.aauw.org/what-we-do/legal-resources/know-your-rights-at-work/workplace-sexual-harassment/employees-guide&r=&t=0).

To report stalking or harassment, call the hotline of the National Center for Victims of Crime at 855-4-VICTIM (855-484-2846) or reach them via online chat (chat.victimconnect.org). Crime victims can also learn about their civil and legal rights at www.victimconnect.org.

To find an appropriate local health facility that is prepared to care for survivors, call the National Sexual Assault Hotline at 800-656-HOPE (4673). You'll be connected to a staff member from a local sexual assault service provider who will explain how to get help and report to law enforcement.

Chapter 10: Online Harassment and Stalking

The Pew Research Center's report on online harassment was published on July 11, 2017, on the organization's website. The Department of Justice periodically updates its statistics. The latest report (https://bjs.gov/content/pub/pdf/svus_rev.pdf) came out in September 2012.

DeleteMe can be found on the Abine website (https://www.abine.com/deleteme/).

CallerSmart also provides a guide on cyberstalking (www.callersmart.com/guides).

FightCyberstalking.org is an online resource providing information on reporting a cyberstalker and online safety tips for social media sites. It offers a tool kit for keeping logs of incidents and communications (in PDF format). The Stalking Resource Center of the National Center for Victims of Crime provides resources on criminal stalking laws by state (https://victimsofcrime.org/our-programs/past-programs/stalking-resource-center/stalking-laws/criminal-stalking-laws-by-state).

A list of states' porn revenge laws can be found at https://www.cybercivilrights.org/revenge-porn-laws/.

Chapter 11: Dodge the Hack—Electronic Security

Take a look at www.securityplanner.org for a user-friendly guide to basic online practices. Security Planner is a project of Citizen Lab, an initiative of the University of Toronto.

The Electronic Frontier Foundation, an international digital rights group, publishes information about tools and holds events around the world. It fields queries and gives updates about vulnerabilities. You can request a speaker at www.eff.org.

CryptoParty (www.cryptoparty.in) is a global movement that holds free events on digital protection. Topics can include encrypted communication, preventing yourself from being tracked while browsing the Web, and general security advice regarding computers and smartphones. You can attend one of its many gatherings, or organize your own.

The MIT Technology Review cites a study by the firm Emsisoft software company that tallied 764 Ransomware attacks on healthcare providers and 89 on educational establishments: https://www.technologyreview.com/f/615002/ransomware-may-have-cost-the-us-more-than-75-billion-in-2019/.

When choosing a VPN, avoid any that log user activity. Opt only for one that is highly regarded in security circles, such as the easy-to-use TunnelBear. Vypr is known as the Cadillac of VPNs for its popularity with the corporate world; it's made by a German company. Activists prefer Private Internet Access. Mullvad, from Sweden, also gets high marks.

Aside from checking if you were a victim of a breach, www.haveibeenpwned.com—"pwned" refers to being compromised—allows you to set up alerts for any possible future breaches. It's free and user-friendly—even for cyberphobics like me.

Suggested camouflage for facial recognition: https://cvdazzle.com/.

Chapter 12: Mental Armor—Emotional Resilience

For a formal definition of PTSD, consult https://www.nimh.nih.gov/health/topics/post-traumatic-stress-disorder-ptsd/index.shtml. A diagnosis includes the following:

Reexperiencing symptoms (flashbacks, intrusive memories, or nightmares);
Avoiding places or thoughts related to the event;
Experiencing arousal and reactivity symptoms (difficulty sleeping, being on edge, quick to anger); and
Having cognitive or mood disorders (e.g., feeling intense guilt or losing hope and interest in activities once found enjoyable).

The Sidran Institute (https://www.sidran.org), for traumatic stress education and advocacy, provides information on hotlines and literature on trauma.

The clinician directory of the International Society for Traumatic Stress Studies (https://www.istss.org/find-a-clinician.aspx) lists various factors to consider when searching for a counselor or mental health professional, such as specialties, populations served, and languages spoken.

The Rebels Project (http://www.therebelsproject.org/) provides support for people impacted by gun violence.

The National Center for PTSD at the National Institute of Mental Health (www.ptsd.va.gov) offers more resources, especially for veterans.

It would be difficult to list all the scholarship that has been done on the link between psychological resilience and eating fruits and vegetables. Two studies leapt out at me:

Shahriar Gharibzadeh, Motaharsadat Hosseini, Saeed Shoar, and Sayed Hoseini, "Depression and Fruit Treatment," *Journal of Neuropsychiatry and Clinical Neurosciences* 22, no. 4 (October 2010): 451–m.e25–451.e25.

S. Mihshahi, A. J. Dobson, and G. D. Mishra, "Fruit and Vegetable Consumption and Prevalence and Incidence of Depressive Symptoms in Mid-age Women: Results from the Australia Longitudinal Study on Women's Health," *European Journal of Clinical Nutrition* 69, no.5 (May 2015), 585–91.

Viktor Frankl, *Man's Search for Meaning*, (New York: Beacon Press, 2006). The book is a profound meditation on Frankl's five years in concentration camps and on what enabled him to cope psychologically.

Conclusion

Author interviews with Albert Bandura, 2018 and 2019. A selected bibliography of Bandura's extensive works appears on his website:https://albertbandura.com/albert-bandura-academic-publications.html.

FORMS

YOUR NAME

Mobile phone and any other numbers

Address

Email

Passwords and PINs for:

Phone

Computer

Bank accounts

Names of important contacts with the same details as above:

Partner

Next of kin

Employer

Doctor

Vet

Lawyer

Financial advisor (should you have one)

Your vital information:

Date of birth

Passport and Social Security numbers

Blood type and any allergies or vital medications like insulin

---

Bank account numbers and passwords

Other account numbers such as credit cards, etc.

Medical and property insurance

Itinerary in case of travel: Details of hotel, airline, vehicles, and departure and arrival times, routes, reservation numbers

---

INDEX

Page numbers of illustrations appear in italics.

ABOUT THE AUTHOR

JUDITH MATLOFF teaches conflict reporting at Columbia's Graduate School of Journalism. She has pioneered safety training seminars for journalists, specifically women, helping hundreds of people feel confident to face an increasingly dangerous world. Her stories about war and violence have appeared in numerous publications, including the *New York Times Magazine*, the *Economist*, the *Los Angeles Times*, and the *Wall Street Journal*. Matloff's work has been supported by the MacArthur Foundation, the Fulbright Scholar Program, the Logan Nonfiction Fellowship, and the Hoover Institution. She lives in New York City with her family.